HOW TO SURVIVE
YOUR HUSBAND'S HEART ATTACK

HOW TO SURVIVE YOUR HUSBAND'S HEART ATTACK

*What You Both Need to Know
to Put Your Lives Back Together*

JOANN STICHMAN

JANE SCHOENBERG

*Produced by Whitehall,
Hadlyme & Smith, Inc.*

David McKay Company, Inc.
NEW YORK

"How to Survive Your Husband's Heart Attack," Chapter 3, by J. Schoenberg and
JoAnn Stichman. Copyright © 1972 by Baywood Publishing Company, New York.
Originally published by *Omega,* Volume 3, Number 2, May 1972. Used with permis-
sion of the publishers.

"Counseling the Coronary Patient on Sexual Activity" by Dr. Reuben Koller, et. al.
Copyright © 1972 by McGraw-Hill, Inc. Published by *Post-Graduate Medicine,* April
1972. Used with permission of the publishers.

But We Were Born Free by Elmer Davis. Copyright © 1952, 1953, 1954 by Elmer Davis.
Published by The Bobbs-Merrill Company, Inc. Used with permission of the publishers.

"Recipes for Fat-Controlled Low Cholesterol Meals" by the American Heart Association. Copyright © 1968, 1972, 1973 by the American Heart Association. Used with
their permission.

Haute Cuisine for Your Heart's Delight by Carol Cutler. Copyright © 1973 by Carol
Cutler. Published by Crown Publishers. Used with permission of the publishers.

Heart Attacks: You Don't Have to Die by Dr. Christiaan Barnard. Copyright © 1972 by
Christiaan Barnard. Published by the Delacorte Press. Used with permission of the
publishers.

Library of Congress Catalog Card Number: 74-76722
ISBN: 0-679-50445-1
MANUFACTURED IN THE UNITED STATES OF AMERICA

To Forrest and Arthur.
And their doctors, Mike Thorner
and Sel Bleifer—for all the obvious reasons.

Foreword

This is an important book written by wives for wives. The experiences related are expressed in words which are refreshingly akin to daily conversation. The book covers the entire spectrum of heart attack experience from the onset—the emergency paramedic attendance, the coronary care unit, the recovery period, home rehabilitation, preventive measures to avoid another attack, and finally the restoration of full participation in marital life and the return to an accustomed occupation.

This is not a book of prohibitions, but rather one of helpful suggestions from two women, each of whom has coped successfully with her husband's heart attack and has met, talked with, and counseled many wives who are faced with the realities of caring for a husband who has survived a heart attack. This book is a communication with real people, covering all of the problems a wife must face and solve. The helpful conversations deal with acceptance of illness; with diet, exercise, sexual activity, and thoughts of divorce; and with the happiness of a wife who has successfully coped with the dangers and realities of an illness with lifetime consequences.

Surely every woman should read this book: for enjoyment, for information, and for the knowledge that forewarning is the best weapon for any battle. The rewards are great, not only in the restoration of a husband's health, but in the revitalization of a happy, successful, lifetime marriage.

George C. Griffith, M.D.,
Master—American College of Physicians
Emeritus Professor of Medicine (Cardiology)
University of Southern California
    School of Medicine

Acknowledgments

This book represents the sum of Heart Wife experiences, thoughts, and emotions we have observed, gathered, or encountered. So, first, we must express our total gratitude to the Heart Wives who gave us so many hours of their time and thought, with so much candor.

Some talked with us as participants in our Heart Wife programs at UCLA Hospital and Cedars-Sinai Medical Center while their husbands were still in the Coronary Care Unit. In theory we were there to help them; in practice we helped each other. But, then, that is what the Heart Wife program is all about.

The debt we owe the women who had already become Heart Wives months or years before we started the program is, if possible, even greater. They generously shared their experiences, even though it meant recalling and reliving some of the most agonizing moments in their lives. We are gratified that the discussions, however painful, were as rewarding, supportive, and helpful for them as they were for the newest Heart Wives, and for us. In the following pages we must sometimes criticize certain actions or attitudes of these women. We ask you to remember this: they freely, candidly, and consciously exposed themselves to criticism *in order to help you avoid the mistakes they made.* That, too, is what Heart Wives are all about. And we cannot think of a more gracious or more touching gift.

Inevitably, people will recognize their own experiences and their own words. But we have purposely omitted names of Heart Wives and changed circumstantial details wherever such changes would do no violence to the instructive point of the experience; so it is unlikely that people who think they recognize other people will be correct. Unlikely, but not impossible. And since the Heart Wives who helped us knew that, it is still another measure of their generosity that they were so willing to help us help you.

There are others to whom we owe deep thanks:

Dr. M. C. Thorner, who has been our mainstay for medical (and general) advice, our instructor, encourager, and friend. He read the manuscript in several versions and improved each one.

Dr. Selwyn Bleifer, especially for his insights and contributions to Chapter 18.

Dr. Norman B. Atkins for his advice and kind patience in helping us understand.

Dr. Kenneth House, especially for his help with Chapters 8 and 12.

Dr. Marvin Goodwin, who helped us understand much more clearly the emotions of children and their reactions.

If errors in medical facts, or interpretation of those facts, have crept into our text it is our fault, not theirs.

We also want to thank:

Dr. Harvey Alpern and his associates on the Coronary Advisory Committee of Cedars-Sinai for their support and direction of the Heart Wife program.

The Department of Medical Social Services at Cedars-Sinai for their many hours of help and patience; especially Nancy Bernstein for her unflagging effort; and the women who so generously give their time, their services, and themselves as volunteers in the program.

The staffs of the Coronary Care Unit and Social Services department at UCLA Hospital, where our program first took shape.

Hermine Lee, whose expertise in nutrition informs much of Chapter 15.

Erna Gallenberg, Director of Patient Relations, and Larry Baum, Director of Community Relations (both at Cedars-Sinai), for their early and continuing help and encouragement.

Charlotte Langley, Unit Supervisor, Vista del Mar Child Care Services, who was the first to say "go ahead," and then patiently taught us how.

Robert Kirsch, who said "keep going"—and helped us do it.

Dr. Richard Kalish, for his help and encouragement—both as a teacher at UCLA and as editor of *Omega*.

Finally, we want to acknowledge formally our gratitude to Andrea Frazier, Reuben Koller, Fred McCuiston, and Annamarie Shaw for contributions that will be obvious as you encounter their names and read what they told us.

Contents

THE HOME

THE
CORONARY CARE
UNIT

CHAPTER

1

Let Us Be
the First to Tell You

Congratulations!

Your husband has survived! What's more, he will continue to survive this heart attack! In the days, weeks, months, and, yes, years ahead, there will be times when you feel this heart attack is going to be the death of you; but it is not going to be the death of him.

How can we be so sure when we don't know you, don't know your husband, don't know anything about his case—and aren't even doctors? When, most likely, your own doctor is unwilling to commit himself much further than to say that everything looks good?

The answer, of course, is . . . we can't. Not for absolutely, positively, 100 percent sure. Even so, we stick by what we said: your husband has survived and will continue to survive this heart attack. And that is neither mindless optimism nor foolish ignorance talking; we know more about you and about your husband's condition than you suppose.

To start with, you would not be reading this book unless your husband had survived up to now. That means he is already in a hospital, hopefully one with a specially equipped Coronary Care Unit, or at least a specially equipped (if not quite so specialized) Intensive Care Unit. And, unless you stopped off on the way to the hospital to pick up a copy of our book (which seems improbable even to *us),* at least twenty-four hours have passed since the start of your husband's heart attack. Actually, it has more likely been a matter of days than of hours. We know that for the first few days when our husbands had heart attacks, the only "reading" we managed was of the eyes and the expressions on the faces of doctors and nurses who had just been with our husbands. You probably feel the same.

So it is safe to assume that a fair number of days have passed since your husband's heart attack. (Given that assumption, you may wonder why we discuss problems, as we soon shall, that a wife generally faces in the first few hours of her husband's heart attack. Because it is important to see why those problems occur and where they can lead, even if it is too late to prevent them. Besides, some other Heart Wife may read about them in time to help you; and now you will be able to help others!)

At any rate, if the attack happened as much as four or five days ago, we know all we need to know about your husband's condition. You see, after three days, or thereabouts, a heart attack has caused all the damage to the heart it is going to cause; certainly all the short-term physical damage. And if your husband has survived that, it is enough to let us assure you that, yes, he will survive this attack. In Chapter 2 we will explain in greater detail exactly why we are so sure. For now, let's leave it at this: he will survive!

Still . . . if we can be so positive and reassuring, why is your husband's doctor so cautious? Is he just being cagey? No. He is just being a doctor, and being positive and reassuring to the patient's wife is not a doctor's job; doing the things that let *us* be positive and reassuring is. Then, too, any doctor knows that any wife in these worrisome circumstances will take positive reassurance as an absolute, "money-back" guarantee, of which there simply are no such things in medicine. If, against all odds, there are complications, the doctor has to look you in the eye. We don't.

Now, we do not mean to sound ominous. But we are hedging, and in a way the doctor cannot possibly do. You may have noticed that we keep saying *"this* heart attack." That is not to say your husband will ever have another. He very well may not. And it is certainly not to say that he will not survive another heart attack. Or another. Or another. Or any number of subsequent attacks. No one knows. But the fact that he has had a heart attack means conditions exist in his arteries (exactly what they are is also explained in Chapter 2) that can lead to other heart attacks. And heart attacks can be fatal.

Knowing that, can you blame the doctor for being more restrained than we are? Would you willingly put yourself in the position of ever having to explain to a distraught wife that her husband did, indeed, survive the first heart attack, as promised, but it was the sudden, million-to-one-against, *second* heart attack that killed him? Of course not. Neither would your husband's doctor. But we do not have to make these nice distinctions to a distraught wife. And while we have no idea of what the actual odds are against your husband having another heart attack so swift and so massive that even the almost miraculous machines, medicines and people of a Coronary Care Unit cannot cope with it, they are so astronomically high that we say again what we said before. Your husband has survived and will survive.

This heart attack.

That is not more hedging. This time "this" means something quite different, something that brings us to the point of this book and the reason for it.

The real problem of a heart attack is not the possibility of dying; it is the much greater probability of living. Because the question immediately comes: living how? What kind of life will it be?

In a curious way it is not really the heart attack that can cause problems affecting the quality of the life your husband and you will lead. You are facing problems today. You will face more tomorrow and the next day and every "next day" of your life. But they are not problems exclusively connected with the particular physical illness called a "heart attack." They are a result of the very human reaction of nearly all patients to certain effects on the body and—more important—on the mind. And, strangely enough, the threat of death is not the most troublesome aspect of a heart attack.

For instance, tuberculosis, typhus, typhoid, and pulmonary pneumonia are all potential killers. But once you are over them, that's that. There is no reason to be any more worried about those diseases than before you got them. Your own life need not be particularly different; your family will not have to make any particular adjustments. You might say those diseases can kill you, but they can't hurt you.

A heart attack is different. There is no "cure." The patient can always have another attack at any time, and there is no sure way to prevent it. But there are things he can do—must do, really—to cut down the chances of another attack. Those things add up to a different sort of life-style for him, his wife, and family. And, even so, there are no guarantees. He can be just as "careful" as you please, do all the right things . . . and still have another attack.

Think what that means to your husband. He has had agonizing pain. He has been in mortal peril. And he knows that he will always run the risk of more pain, and sudden death. He wants to live, though, so he will do everything he can to increase his chances. But what does that mean? He does not know if he will be able to work as hard or as well as he did before. Or at all. He may have to change jobs if he was doing heavy, strenuous work. He may not be able to earn the money he did before. He will have to stop smoking, watch his weight, give up many foods and activities he used to enjoy.

Faced with all that, any man has to be apprehensive, anxious, and depressed about his future. And hostile. Why him? Why should he have been the one to be stricken? He will take that hostility out on everyone around him.

In short, we are talking about a personality and behavior change, as well as a distinct change in life-style.

How long must you expect these changes to continue? For the rest of your life. Remember what we said before: the heart attack showed that conditions exist that can (not will, can) cause another; and as long as a man lives with that knowledge, there will be problems.

A friend of ours suggested that the motto for this book should be the one you have surely seen on little placards in gift shops: "Today is the first day of the rest of your life." She meant that the life you lead as a Heart Wife is continuing and, in effect, is a new sort of life, with new sorts of problems, new challenges, and new rewards. That is true; and it is a valuable insight. But the phrase, itself, suggests a rather dangerous way of thinking for a Heart Wife. It suggests that, somehow, each new day can be a clean slate; that you can always start over, without regard for the past. And that is not true for you. Today, tomorrow, and every day from now on, will start with the *fact* of your husband's heart attack.

The life this book describes is not a brief interlude between the first pains in your husband's chest and some undefined, yet definite, day to come when he will be "over" his heart attack and everything will go back to what it was. Our purpose is to help you solve the problems we know you will face. Today, tomorrow, twenty years from now. But not so you can "go back" to a life in which the problems peculiar to the wife and family of a heart patient do not exist. Because you will never live that sort of life again, not while your husband lives. What you will read about here is a way of life—in many ways, perhaps most ways, a richer and more sensible life than you ever led before. But a different life. With different problems.

You will not face every one of the problems we examine in this book (we certainly hope not, anyway!). We have tried to present all of the different kinds of problems that we have come across, both in our own cases and the hundreds of cases we and our Heart Wife Counselors have handled since we began the Heart Wife program (which, incidentally, is described in Chapter 3). The problems are discussed in the order we have found they typically come up during each stage of recovery. Every person's own problems may vary slightly with the patient's or wife's particular situation or personality. If you find that details of your problems are different or missing from the ones discussed, don't be concerned. This book is a sort of map for the trip you are taking through country that is very strange to you, very frightening, with many wrong turns, many pitfalls, and very few road signs. Don't worry if the map does not show every bend in the road. The main intersections are there. The blind alleys and detours around rough stretches are all clearly marked, and after all, that is what a map is for.

We cannot give you exact solutions to all your problems; human problems don't have exact solutions, and there are no magic recipes for solving them. But we can make you aware of problems before they come up, of problems that can develop without your noticing; and we can show you how other women have successfully handled those problems.

It might be a good idea to let your close friends and relatives read this book. No one who has not gone through it can really know what you are experiencing. But this book may help them understand. They want to help; they will surely be able to help you, your husband, and your family better if they understand what the problems are. That is also true for your husband, and for the same reason: you can help each other better if you understand each other's problems.

But a word of caution. Do not let your husband see this book until you have talked about it with his doctor. We will say this again and again; we cannot say it too often or stress it too much. Do not let anyone (including us) give you any advice (including what you find in this book) that directly affects your husband unless his doctor approves. The doctor is the only person qualified to approve any kind of treatment, physical or mental, for your husband. With very few exceptions, the advice or suggestions we will make are for you. They will benefit your husband because they help you make the atmosphere in which he will recover more pleasant; but they do not directly affect him. We are qualified to offer suggestions to you, qualified in a way even your doctor is not, unless your doctor happens to be a woman whose husband has had a heart attack. But we are not qualified to suggest anything to, or for, your husband. And neither is anyone else, except his doctor!

Perhaps the most valuable thing that this book can tell you is that you are not strange or awful for having some of the thoughts and emotions you have and will have. You are not unique in the problems you have and will have; others have had them, solved them, and are now going to help you solve them. You are not alone.

CHAPTER

2

His Survival—And Yours

His Survival

Your husband's doctor has probably explained what causes a heart attack. Or tried to, anyway. Your mind was on other matters.

Almost every Heart Wife feels the same. A nurse who is part of one of the country's leading open-heart surgery teams told us, "I've noticed that the wives talking to the doctor just before an operation—finding out what is going to happen—just *do not hear*. They hear, 'Your husband should probably have an operation, because if he doesn't have one, there's a very good chance that he might die.' But, beyond that . . . they've heard as much as they can handle."

Well, if we are not apt to hear a doctor explaining fairly dramatic surgery that's about to take place, we certainly are not going to hang on his every syllable about a heart attack that has already occurred. And the truth is, most of us start with only the dimmest notion of what happens to cause a heart attack, why it happens, and what happens next. That may seem strange, considering how much we hear about heart disease these days. But nearly everything we hear is directed toward warning us of "danger signals," telling us how to avoid heart attacks, and selling us polyunsaturated margarine. Which leaves us fairly blank when it comes to actual knowledge. As one Heart Wife put it, "The doctor came out of the Coronary Care Unit and told me it was an 'infarction.' My God! It was the first time, I think, I ever heard the word."

Does it make any difference whether or not you understand the vocabulary and mechanics of a failing heart? Yes, it does. In fact, it makes a world of difference. Unless you know what causes a heart attack, how can you help prevent another? What's more, unless you understand what the doctor tells you about heart attacks, many of the other things he tells you will not make much sense, including what he tells you about your husband's chances of living and the things you can do to improve those chances.

Start with that word "infarction." What is it, how does it happen, and what has it done to your husband's heart?

The heart, of course, pumps blood around the body. It contracts, forcing the blood inside it out through the body's largest artery, the aorta, to carry oxygen to tissue throughout the body.

If anything cuts off the flow of blood—a tourniquet around your leg, for instance—no blood can get to the tissue below the tourniquet. No blood means no oxygen. And without oxygen, tissue dies.

If the supply of blood is not completely shut off, tissue may simply get too little oxygen. It does not die, it just gets what we might call sick. Sit with your legs firmly crossed for a while and there will be pressure on the femoral artery; put enough pressure on long enough and tissue below the pressure point will "fall asleep." This is tissue's way of telling you that it needs more oxygen and that you had better do something about it before things get serious.

The heart is tissue, too—muscle tissue, mostly. And it needs a great deal more blood than most other tissue in the body because it works harder and burns up more oxygen.

So, sensibly enough, the heart feeds itself first. It has its own, special arteries, called the "coronary arteries," which are the first to branch off from the aorta. Each of these two coronary arteries is about four to five inches long, with many tiny branches that reach all parts of the heart. At its widest, the opening in a coronary artery is about one-eighth of an inch across. That does not sound very wide, but it is actually more than wide enough. And the word "more" is extremely important. A fatty substance called "cholesterol" tends to cling to the inner lining of all arteries—the coronaries, unfortunately, included. As cholesterol builds up, it irritates the lining of an artery. The body's natural reaction is to cover over anything irritating its tissue with tough, fibrous scar tissue. The trouble is, more cholestrol keeps accumulating, then more fiber, layer on layer, while the arterial opening keeps getting narrower.

Whenever a coronary artery gets so clogged that not enough blood gets through to give the heart tissue the oxygen it needs, there is trouble.

The artery may be completely closed. Sometimes the "plaque"—which is what doctors call the hardened cholesterol and fibrous scar tissue—is ruptured. The place where the rupture took place swells, the way a cut on your finger becomes puffy, and it blocks what was left of the opening in the already narrowed artery. Either way—totally blocked or just not open enough—the heart tissue usually fed by that artery is starved and dies. That is called an "infarction."

Not all of the heart is affected, only the tissue "downstream" from where the coronary artery is blocked. How serious the heart attack is depends on what part of the heart, and how much of it, is involved. If only a very small branch of the artery is blocked, the victim may not even know he has had a heart attack; he will think it is indigestion, or some such trivial disagreement between nature and his system.

But if enough of the heart is affected and not able to keep beating, the attack is almost immediately fatal.

Between those extremes, there are all degrees of severity,

from mild to massive. There is plenty that can be done to save the patient even at the outer limits of massive attacks.

Nothing can "cure" the attack or unclog the arteries. No medicine, anyway. Nature is another matter. Given time, the heart will heal itself. Scar tissue forms on the infarction; new branches of the coronary arteries grow into the area and, through "collateral circulation," take over the job of the blocked branch. What a doctor does, with the help of machines and medicines, nurses and technicians, is to give the heart the time it needs. Christiaan Barnard, a doctor whose name is associated with more dramatic heart treatments, outlined the typical time-gaining measures in his book *Heart Attack: You Don't Have to Die* (Delacorte, 1972).

> Drugs are given to alleviate the pain and fear that contribute to the shock. The air that the patient breathes is enriched with oxygen to raise the concentration of this vital element in whatever blood is reaching the ischemic muscle. Sodium bicarbonate is given intravenously to neutralize the lactic acid that accumulates as a result of poor blood flow through the tissues, and cardiac stimulants and drugs to elevate the blood pressure are cautiously administered. All of these procedures are designed to arrest the spread of the area of cell death and to carry the patient through the crisis—to buy just that little bit of time that is required for the acute phase to pass and for spontaneous recovery to occur.

The trouble is that right after an attack the heart is badly shaken and weakened. But it still has to do its job; it has to keep pumping blood to the rest of the body. Since part of it is not functioning, though, it is working inefficiently. The timing of its beating may be off, a problem called "arrhythmia." In a Coronary Care Unit, to quote an American Heart Association pamphlet, "that isn't necessarily dangerous." Arrhythmia can be corrected, by proper care, even before it really gets started. Outside of a hospital, arrhythmia is extremely dangerous. And since about 90 percent of heart patients experience some sort of arrhythmia, the need for getting to a hospital fast is obvious. To quote Dr. Barnard again:

> . . . of all patients dying as a result of heart attacks, 70 percent die before receiving any medical attention at all and 60 percent die within the first hour of the attack. All the evidence indicates that a majority of these deaths are due to arrhythmias and are hence preventable.

Just in case you read that too fast, let us emphasize the words ". . . of all patients dying." It does not mean that 70 percent of all heart attack victims die; just that of those who *do* die, 70 percent receive no treatment.

But, as we said in the first chapter, we can assume that your husband is already in a hospital. So what are his chances? Well, as soon as he got there, they went up sharply. If he is in a Coronary Care Unit, his chances are even better (about 3,000 of the 7,000 hospitals in the United States have Coronary Care Units; but the number keeps growing; and most of the others have Intensive Care Units). According to the Heart Association, 40 percent of first heart attacks are fatal—BUT the majority of those deaths occur in the first hour. In 1966, 50 percent of all first-attack deaths came within one hour. (Dr. Barnard's 60 percent includes all attacks, not just the first.) That figure has now gone up to 65 percent largely because of the increasing number and sophistication of Coronary Care Units. It does not mean that more people die in the first hour; it means that fewer people who make it to a hospital die. In fact, the Heart Association says, "It has been established that in-hospital death rates following heart attacks can be reduced by about 30 percent if the patient gets optimum coronary care . . ."

So one hour after his attack, your husband's statistical chances double if it is his first attack.

The next sharp increase in his chances to survive comes four hours after the attack. That's because of one particularly dangerous kind of arrhythmia, called "ventricular fibrillation." Quoting the Heart Association again, that "is about twenty-five times more likely to occur during the first four hours from the start of the attack than during the ensuing twenty-four hours."

If we called his chances "good" after one hour, they have to be called distinctly "better" after four hours. Seventy-two hours after the attack they are very good indeed. By then, almost everything bad that can happen to his heart has already happened—for now, at any rate. That is why patients are generally released from a Coronary Care Unit after five days to a week (although, as we will explain in later chapters, longer stays in the CCU or in the hospital do not necessarily mean that one individual is in worse shape than another). Seven days after the attack, your husband's chances are, to say the least, excellent.

Finally, after six weeks, if he dies from a heart attack, it is not going to be this one.

Why Did It Happen

Now that we have your husband well on his way to recovery from his heart attack, let's see what caused it. How did that fatty substance, cholesterol, build up in the first place?

Cholesterol is manufactured by each person's liver—but not, ironically, from fatty substance. However, if there is a lot of fat in the diet, and if a person is overweight, the cholesterol he eats, added to his natural cholesterol, is more than his body can burn off.

It is almost exactly the same process that results in a person gaining weight when he eats more than his body needs in the way of calories. Except that instead of merely gathering together as body fat, excess cholesterol fat enters the bloodstream and tends to cling to the walls of all arteries. This, in general, is called atherosclerosis—"hardening of the arteries." So diet is clearly one important factor in bringing on heart attacks.

Heredity is another. Heart disease seems to run in families; some people are born with a tendency to have too much cholesterol in the blood and clogging their arteries. And there is nothing that can be done about it.

A third factor is tension. Again for reasons doctors cannot ascertain, tension seems to increase cholesterol levels in the blood.

If the buildup of cholesterol in the arteries goes on long enough, the heart attack will just happen. But there are things that can hurry it along. Remember that the heart is a muscle. Like any other muscle in the body, it is strengthened by exercise and becomes "flabby" when not exercised. Of course, the heart is always "exercising." However, its regular rate of beating is not enough to make it stronger. And if your husband's job involved mostly sitting, if his hobbies and leisure did not involve much exertion, his heart very seldom beat much faster than its usual rate. Meanwhile, fatty deposits were building up in the coronary arteries, and parts of his heart had to get by with less and less blood. So his heart's ability to cope with any sudden increase in beating rate was steadily going down. If something did make his heart beat much faster, part of the muscle would not get enough oxygen to do its share of the unaccustomed extra work. What's more, the extra effort and extra action of faster beating (with the heart contracting more sharply and rapidly than usual) can rupture the plaque, causing sudden blocking of the artery.

Now you know why so many heart attacks take place on golf courses, tennis courts, and the like. But the extra exertion can be mental, as well as physical. That is especially true if there is a sudden incident causing extreme anger or fear, or tooth-grinding tenseness. The heart beats a tattoo, the blood pressure soars . . . and that's it.

High blood pressure itself (called "hypertension") can also be a significant contributing factor, and is often associated with heart disease. That is one reason why smoking is out for heart patients. Like violent exercise and tension, it increases the heart rate, raises blood pressure, and makes its own special, nasty contribution by constricting blood vessels; heart tissue that is not getting enough blood anyway gets even less through tightened, nicotine-constricted vessels.

Which of the long-range causes clogged your husband's arteries? Which of the immediate causes made his heart attack happen just when it did? In all likelihood, even your doctor is not certain. He may have strong suspicions; but it is nearly impossible to be sure in any particular case. As in any mystery, there are several suspects, each perfectly plausible.

Is it tension? Well, soldiers in combat must be pretty tense. So during the Korean War, army doctors performed autopsies on 300 soldiers who had been killed in action. The average age of the men was just over twenty-two years—but more than three-quarters of them had some heart disease, ranging from the early stages of clogging to complete closing of branch arteries.

Was tension the villain? Not necessarily. Because autopsies were performed on Chinese soldiers, too. They were obviously under the same stress, but there was almost no sign of heart disease among them.

Also consider the studies conducted among prisoners who survived Nazi concentration camps, and among citizens of Stalingrad, a city under continual siege for over two years. Those people had lived through experiences just as nerve-wracking as combat—for a lot longer. Yet there was virtually no heart disease among them!

However, these studies considered another factor: diet. Our soldiers ate foods high in fat content, while the Chinese soldiers ate very few fatty foods. The prisoners and the people of Stalingrad ate practically nothing (many starved to death), certainly not much meat, and no dairy products at all. Autopsies on those who died shortly after their terrifying experience was over showed that fatty deposits in the coronary arteries had been absorbed by the body, which needed every ounce of fat available to it. Six months after the war, there were heart attacks in Stalingrad and among the ex-prisoners once again. And the

coronary disease rate in these groups was soon back to prewar
levels.

Then the most important factor in heart attacks must be diet,
right? Well . . . doctors surely feel that it is vital. But how about
the results of a survey made among some 31,000 employees of
the London Transport Authority? Conductors on double-
decker buses had significantly less heart disease than did the rest
of the men, considered as a whole, or considered as part of three
other job categories: drivers of the double-deckers, drivers of
single-deck buses, and conductors on single-deckers.

All these men must have had pretty much the same sort of
diet. It is true that the double-decker conductors were under
less strain than their drivers; but no less than conductors on
single-deckers. In fact, the only real difference among the
31,000 was that the low-coronary-disease group got more
exercise than the others. They were tramping up and down the
stairs of their double-deckers all day long. Drivers sit; single-
decker conductors walk aisles, but have no stairs to climb. So
you might conclude that the key element in a heart attack is how
much regular exercise you get.

That seems to be confirmed by a survey conducted by two
teams of doctors—one in Boston, the other in Dublin. They
studied 575 pairs of brothers. One of each pair had emigrated as
a young man to the Boston area; the other brother stayed in
Ireland. The results, after nine years of study, were amazing.
The Irishmen, as a group, have far less heart disease than their
transplanted American brothers, even though the Irish brothers
eat from 400 to 500 calories a day *more,* including a substantially
higher percentage of animal fats, rich in the "dreaded"
cholesterol! BUT—and a big one it is!—they get way more
physical exercise.

Does that settle it? It does not.

A similar study was conducted in Sweden, involving thirty-
two pairs of identical twins, only one of whom had had a heart
attack. After exhaustive testing, the significant difference

between the pairs was that those twins who had suffered heart attacks worked harder (though not at physical labor), relaxed less, had more personal, home, and business problems, and in general enjoyed life less.

That adds up to . . . tension. And tension brings us right back where we started.

But it isn't necessary to consider these surveys separately. Taken altogether, they do let us form a conclusive answer. Is the real cause of heart disease bad diet? Lack of exercise? Tension? The answer is . . . "yes"!

In short, there is no one definite cause; there are many contributing causes. Any or all of them may be involved in a particular case. Any or all may cause a particular heart attack. Even more important, correcting any or all of these may be the key to avoiding another attack. But which? Since no one can be sure, all of these factors must be taken into account for the rest of the patient's life.

Now you can see why you must understand what a heart attack is and what can cause it. It is not humanly possible for your husband's doctor to give instructions covering every single area of potential risk. He needs your informed cooperation (and, of course, your husband's, too) in recognizing problems when they come up and in doing something about them. But you cannot help provide solutions until you know what the problems are. Once you do, you are prepared to help achieve your husband's survival. And your own.

Your Survival

"Her survival? *He's* the one in danger." That, or something like it, was said by several people we have talked to about the problems a Heart Wife faces. No one who felt that way, however, was either a heart patient or a patient's wife. They know your survival is not all that clear-cut or sure. We are not talking about "dying of a broken heart," or anything like that; we are not talking about dying at all. But there is a distinct danger that you—just as you are, a wife (with all that means), mother, and woman—that the real you may not survive.

For instance, if you become a nursemaid to your husband, you are not going to survive as a wife; no one can be both. If you get so wrapped up in your own needs, problems, and fears that you cannot cope with those of your children, if you simply give up and become a little girl, yourself, hoping for someone to take care of you, you are not going to survive as a mother. If you cannot adjust to the changes in him and in your life-style, if you make his recovery harder, you may become a widow, or a divorcee, or just a singularly unhappy person trudging through a dead marriage. In any case, your failure will make it very hard for you to survive as a woman.

Helping you survive as you are is what this book is all about.

Your survival depends on a number of things. The relatively simple part involves coping with the routine details of your household and your life, both while he is in the hospital and when he comes home. We say they are "relatively" simple because we can help you directly with specific suggestions for coping with these details that reflect the experiences of many Heart Wives. They have been through it; they stumbled over problems, picked their way along with trial-and-error solutions. Their experience can help you find the less rocky paths.

One thing is central to your survival: your attitude about what has happened.

First, you must realize it *has* happened. We mean it! "Denial" is the term doctors use to describe a reaction to serious illness that is so common they almost look for it. In reporting on their study of the psychological reaction of fifty heart patients to treatment in the Coronary Care Unit of Massachusetts General Hospital, three psychiatrists said this:

> The defense mechanism of denial is defined as the conscious or unconscious repudiation of part or all of the total available meaning of an event to allay fear, anxiety, or other unpleasant

effects. The term "major denial" is used to describe patients who stated unequivocally that they felt no fear at any time throughout their hospital stay; twenty out of the fifty examined were in this group . . .

That means that two out of five simply ignored the fact that they had a potentially fatal illness. If you ignore it, will it go away? The doctors also said that another twenty-six patients had shown "partial denial." They found that it does not go away and that you cannot really ignore it with any great conviction. Even so, many are willing to try.

And patients are not the only ones. We have found that some women we counsel are not ready to face the *fact* of heart attack. They hope if they sort of "pretend" to themselves and their families that nothing is wrong and nothing has changed, maybe something good will happen. Maybe it's a mistake; maybe someone will invent a miracle drug, or just perform a miracle. Maybe *anything*, just so their husbands and families—and they, themselves—will be spared the consequences that relentlessly follow serious illness.

But something has happened. There has been an event in your life that is absolutely unchangeable, with irreversible effects. No doctor, no drug, no operation—nothing on earth—can possibly change the fact that your husband has had a heart attack. If he had broken his leg, there would be no question about it. You know that nothing can "unbreak" the bone. Well, nothing can "unattack" your husband's heart. From the moment he had the attack throughout the rest of his life (which can very possibly be rich, full, and long), he will be someone with "a heart condition." *That will never change.*

A heart attack is a fact, an unchangeable fact with certain consequences that inescapably must be faced.

Your husband will have to lead a somewhat (at the very least) different sort of life from now on. You will also have to lead a different sort of life. Not better, necessarily. Not worse, necessarily. But necessarily different.

Some women's reaction to this inevitable difference in their lives is self-pity. We hope they find comfort or even pleasure from it, because that is most likely the only comfort and pleasure in store for them. And there is a good reason.

You play the key role in your husband's recovery. You set the tone and atmosphere. Your attitude toward the adjustments you must make directly affect the adjustments he must make. The success with which he recovers and adjusts will be a direct measure of how well you do your job; no matter how great (or small) a part you played in shaping your family's life before, you will play a much greater, much more vital part now.

What you do and how you act, now and for the months to come, will be reflected in how happily you live for years to come. In other, older words that should have a new and special poignancy for all Heart Wives, "As ye sow, so shall ye reap."

Self-pity is just another, slightly fancier, form of denial. A woman can wrap her pity around herself, cozy, comforting, and warm, shutting out the reality of the many things that must be done, paralyzed by the enormity of the misfortune she keeps telling herself has come to her, undeserved and unalterable. She pities herself and does nothing more. After all, what can she do in the face of such disaster? Soon the things she has not done result in her becoming a true object of everyone's pity.

Don't let that be you. Don't deny—in any way—the fact of your husband's illness. Take it as a cue to get on with what must be done, not as a tragedy to be helplessly mourned or an imposition to be revenged. You will cope. And, because you do, you will find that the necessary difference in your life can just as easily be "good-different" as "bad-different." That is because the things you must do eventually center on accommodating your life, your family, and your home to the fact of your husband's heart attack. Do the right things, set a helpful tone for his recovery, an encouraging atmosphere for his adjustment, and you will automatically be doing the things that help you survive. What's more, they are the things that will help make sure he literally survives—continues to live, recover, and grow stronger. And at the same time, help him survive—in the sense that you are surviving—as the man you love and married.

You will not "live to bless the day he had a heart attack" or any such nonsense. Your feelings about it cannot make a particle of difference, so do not waste time blessing—or cursing—an irreversible fact. The day of his heart attack and the days before no longer matter. The days since are your concern. And you may have reason to find most of them a blessing. It's up to you.

CHAPTER

3

Why You Need Help

There is a recurrent theme in nearly every talk we have with Heart Wives. It is reflected in what one woman told us some twelve years later about her reaction to the news that her husband had had a heart attack:

> It was unbelievable! I was twenty-nine, with two babies. I just couldn't believe that it would be possible. I mean, he had been a very, very healthy guy!

Of course, twelve years is a long time. Did she remember it right? Here is what another woman told us just ten days after her husband's heart attack:

> I couldn't believe it! I thought, "Well, there just has to be a mistake. I just spoke to him a couple of hours ago on the phone!"

Twelve years or ten days, the most vivid recollection is one of unbelief. Not *dis*belief—thinking the doctor is not telling the truth or has made a mistake—just inability to believe that such a thing could be true. A cardiac nurse told us she hears almost the identical lament from nearly every new Heart Wife:

> They'll say, "But he's *been* on a low-cholesterol diet. We've *always* avoided meat and eggs."

Or, "But he's been healthy all his life. He works out at the gym three times a week. Look how healthy he is!"

I don't think they want answers. They just want to be able to say the things that are bothering them: "Why did this happen to *him?* He's forty-six years old and he's always taken care of himself."

You know!

Yes, we know. And we imagine you know, too. You have just been there, yourself. From the moment you realized your husband had a heart attack you were operating in a state of shock. It is a weird, frightening state of mind where nothing seems real, nothing seems believable.

You look like someone in shock and act that way, too. Ask anyone who saw you. Or, as we did, ask someone who sees more Heart Wives, day-in and day-out, than the busiest cardiologist.

Fred McCuiston is a paramedic with the Los Angeles City Fire Department Rescue Squad. He was given special medical training in emergency life-sustaining techniques at UCLA, one of a growing number of paramedic training centers. To Fred's mind, there is no question about the state you were in:

About half the time, on a cardiac case, the wife's there. And just going by looks, if you didn't know he's the one you got the call for, you'd probably treat *her* first.

She's so worried and anxious she really doesn't know what she's saying or doing.

For instance, we used to find that a woman would dial the operator and ask for an ambulance for her husband, then hang up and forget to give an address or a name. It happened enough so that they had to change the system. Now it's the first thing the operator asks.

And when we're all set to go, the wife will want to accompany her husband to the hospital. But she'll ask us to wait so she can get everything she needs together.

Of course, we can't. We tell her it's essential that we get her husband to the hospital at once. And we would prefer that she take a cab instead of driving herself. She's in no shape to be behind a wheel!

If the portrait seems exaggerated, remember that Fred sees you with the totally absorbed tunnel vision of a specialist. His specialty is keeping people alive while he rushes them to a hospital. To his mind you did your part when you called for help. From then on you are only in the way. Not that he blames you or is unsympathetic, it's just that he does not think you can help yourself, let alone anyone else!

> Often, when we're all set to leave, a woman will say something to her husband, "Charles, I think you're a little too heavy for them." And she'll want to help us take him down the stairs.
> We don't need this! If we need help, we can always get it. But women at a time like that . . . ? [*he shrugs with the sort of "what're-you-gonna-do" smile that women's lib could use on a recruiting poster.*]
> They think that is helping. It's the only way they can make themselves feel that they have tried to do something.

Next to the heart attack itself, your crushing sense of helplessness is probably the greatest element of your shock. As one Heart Wife said,

> You're just completely in everybody's hands. That's the worst feeling—that you're powerless to do anything.

It is the worst, but not by much. All the events, sights, sounds, and people that attend a heart attack conspire to put you in shock and keep you there, dazed and disoriented from the very first.

If you were with your husband at the time of the attack, you had the sight and sound of his pain and peril, knowing there was nothing you could do about either. Then there was the ambulance, the oxygen, the flashing lights and siren, the traffic signals ignored. Or maybe a frenzied car ride—with you at the wheel. Or there was that grim phone call with the message, and not knowing whether he was still alive until you reached the hospital. Not that it ends once you are at the hospital. Now there is the CCU, with your husband plugged into monstrous-looking machines and tubes and bottles (never mind that they are saving his life: knowing that cannot diminish their graphic demonstration of how sick he is).

Furthermore, it is not until your husband gets to the hospital that you discover what helplessness *really* feels like. Compared to your role in the Coronary Care Unit, you were practically the key member of the rescue team. In a pinch you actually *could* take a corner of the stretcher (in point of fact, Fred would probably show the more distressing signs of cardiac arrest, himself, if you so much as touched it; but at least you *could* have helped). At the hospital you are strictly excess baggage.

To rub it in, there is a positive frenzy of helpfulness going on all around. Your husband is an island of need entirely surrounded by competent professionals doing the one thing on earth you would like to do: help him. They are; you are not. Indeed, you are the only one in sight who is not doing a thing to help him. The staff's calm efficiency is a reproach to your distraught helplessness. Even the rigid time limit for visiting in a CCU—five minutes an hour—even that shows what the starchy professionals think of you; you are simply in the way.

None of this is calculated to build your confidence.

The reaction of a woman at one of the first Heart Wife group meetings we held at UCLA Hospital says it all. She came into the meeting very flustered, almost in tears, then sat and glared in the general direction of the CCU. Up to then she had been remarkable for her easy acceptance, her placid conviction that everything was going to be all right because it's "all in God's hands." We asked her what was troubling her. Evidently, someone besides God had been taking a good deal too much of a hand in things for her taste:

> I was going in to see my husband, and the doctor was there. He said to me, "Would you mind waiting outside a minute? I've got to talk with your husband."
> What secrets do they have that his own wife can't hear?

Then her fears and hurts and resentments came pouring out. She told of her "suspicions" that she was "being closed out of this thing."

Another Heart Wife started feeling "closed out" on the way to the hospital in the ambulance:

> They wouldn't let me get in back with him, which upset me terribly, because I didn't know what was going to happen.
>
> I sat in front with the driver. But I could see they were talking back there. And I kept thinking, "They won't let me back there, but they keep making him talk! He should be resting, not talking!"
>
> I found out later that the attendant was getting my husband's history. But at the time. . . !

The fact is that the words and acts of the doctors, nurses, and other hospital personnel can materially add to your feelings of being helpless and useless, of being inadequate to the point of idiocy—finally, of being guilty for not being able to surmount both the feeling and fact of your shocked paralysis. They are wrapped up in their concern for the patient and are likely to be too busy to be tactful, understanding, and supportive in their dealings with you. And some may simply have brusque, abrasive personalities.

One Heart Wife told us how she had rushed up to meet the cardiologist as he came out of the CCU after seeing her husband for the first time. He told her it was almost definitely a heart attack but that her husband would be all right. Practically radiating relief, she asked what she could do to help. "Get that fat off him," the doctor snapped, and bustled out of the room, leaving her feeling "like a naughty little girl who was too dumb, or too lazy, to have done her duty."

Where do experiences like that leave you? In shock. What's more, you do nothing to reduce the shock to your mind or system. You get little or no sleep, practically no food. And for the first few days you may be living with that most exquisite torment, false hope. The majority of heart attacks do not show up on the only two unequivocal tests—electrocardiogram and enzyme test—for seventy-two hours or so. All you can do is hope and fear. Mostly fear. But even the frail, intermittent hope is clouded by the thought that, well, if not his heart . . . what? That kind of anxiety does not help any.

And through it all, you are convinced that nobody can help you, that nobody knows or can understand what it is like. You know you cannot help your husband. And you are equally sure no one can help you, if only because no one can possibly know what you are going through. Your specific problems and emotions both seem unimaginable for anyone who has not experienced them; you are positive you could not have imagined what it was like beforehand. Either you have "been there" or you have not. If not, those problems defy thought and reason. There just is not much in the way of practical advice or even meaningful comfort an "outsider" can offer. As one Heart Wife said:

> Oh! Are you by yourself! There's a lot of action going on. Friends come and sit and try to tell you everything's going to be all right; but they don't *know*. And they don't know anything else to say.
>
> Then there are lots of hospital people running in and out. But everybody seems to be really indifferent to you.
>
> I guess they're not, *really*. But they're busy doing whatever they're doing and they simply don't notice. Maybe it's just that they're so used to seeing us sit there.
>
> But . . . oh! Are you ever by yourself!

That means having no one who knows what problems you are facing and what problems are coming, no one who could perhaps help you solve them. Worse still, there is no one to give you the kind of sympathy you want and need. Informed sympathy. Sympathy reflecting some true understanding of just how awful the problems are. People who do not truly know what they are sympathizing with really are not much comfort. Their sympathy, no matter how sincere, just does not do justice to the misfortune!

A psychiatrist we talked with put it this way:

It's the difference between having your house destroyed in something like the Wilkes Barre flood or Malibu fire or a Florida hurricane—and having a freak accident hit you without touching your neighbors' homes. Objectively, the loss is the same. But there's a comfort in sharing calamity. The people around you know how you feel, because they feel exactly the same. So, with them you can talk with the heart, not just the mind.

"Heart-to-heart" is the indispensable dialogue for you right now. Yet there you are, with no one who understands, with either head or heart. You have no idea where to find someone who understands. You might not even realize you need such a person. After all, the reason you feel so alone is because you do not know it is possible for anyone else to have the slightest inkling of how you feel. And you can scarcely be expected to go looking for someone to warn you of problems that have not occurred yet. So all you can do is sit. And worry.

No wonder you are in shock. No wonder you need help. That is why we started the Heart Wife Program, and why we wrote this book. In that order. We began the Heart Wife program at UCLA Hospital on a fairly informal, part-time basis. Almost at once it was requiring more and more time and organization. Very soon, we received a private grant to establish the program at Cedars-Sinai Medical Center, specifically in the Coronary Unit at Cedars of Lebanon Hospital, as part of the Social Services Department, and under the direction of Dr. Harvey L. Alpern, of the Coronary Advisory Committee at Cedars.

Right now, we are in full operation at Cedars, with several volunteer Heart Wives helping with the counseling, and we are beginning to receive inquiries about the formation of Heart Wife programs at other hospitals.

The program is growing; but your need is *now*.

You Are Not Alone

That is the basic message of the Heart Wives program and of this book. You are *not* alone.

How does the program work? What kind of help does it offer?

At the first practical moment, with the permission, or at the request, of the patient's doctor, the CCU charge nurse introduces a new Heart Wife to a Heart Wife Counselor. Let's say the new Heart Wife is you.

At first, all you probably want to talk about is how unbelievable it is, and to tell us exactly what happened from the moment your husband said he did not feel well until he got to the hospital. What you mostly want us to tell you is how well our husbands are doing, as reassurance that husbands do recover.

But even at first we can help in some practical ways. We can make you aware, or remind you, of things that must be taken care of right away, such as thinking through who should be told about your husband's condition, what they should be told, and who should tell them. Equally important, we can discuss who should perhaps not be told, and why not.

Of course, if you want to know more about your husband's condition, we will answer your questions, or get someone who can answer them. A cardiologist, a cardiac nurse, a dietician, a social-services worker. But very few women can focus on much long-term information those first days.

When your husband is out of the CCU—that is when you start wanting solid information. Now is the time to review the possibly slapdash arrangements you barely had time to improvise for your family, your home, and yourself. Now is when you are ready to find out what a heart attack is and what its implications are for the future. You attend weekly Heart Wife meetings, where a cardiologist and/or a cardiac nurse, a dietician, and a psychiatric social-services worker meet informally with Heart Wives whose husbands are still in the hospital.

It is impossible to overstate the importance and value of these professionals' presence at the weekly meetings. Just knowing they are available to answer questions helps build your confidence that you are doing everything you can to prepare yourself for problems in your husband's recovery and your family's adjustment. What's more, the meetings let professionals use their skill and expertise in the most efficient way. Each is of maximum service to a maximum number of heart-patient families with a minimum of time, fuss, and bother.

The two inseparable ingredients of the meetings are discussion and questions. The only rule is, "Let it all hang out." One Heart Wife's full and frank discussion will encourage another to ask questions she otherwise might never "remember" or "dare" to ask. You hear about problems that have not come up for you yet. You get a fix on possible ways of handling them if they do. And you can call on professionals for help in finding solutions.

Our role at these meetings depends on how spontaneous any group is at the time. If everyone is tight-lipped, we get things started by talking about our own experiences during the hospital stage, asking the professionals questions that occur to nearly all Heart Wives, even if they are not ready to ask on their own. Like how to limit friends' and relatives' visiting time without offending them; organizing the household; what to tell the children; arranging transportation; and general problems of morale—yours, your husband's, the children's, maybe even the doctor's!

Usually, though, we are just members of the group—but with the advantage of hindsight, knowing what we wished we had known when we were going through the same experience.

These meetings are the most important part of the program during the hospital stage of recovery. However, we are available, both at the hospital and over the phone, to sit and talk over problems you would rather not air at a meeting.

All of this is in preparation for the next, never-ending phase of recovery that starts when your husband leaves the hospital for home:

You are as ready as you can be. The cardiologist has gone into the general medical aspects of heart recovery, so you know what to expect; the nurse has explained how to make bed rest most comfortable; the dietician has given you ideas for minimizing the clash between how your family used to eat and how a heart patient must be fed; you also have a good grasp of what the psychological problems usually are for a man recovering from a heart attack.

Even so, you and your husband still need help. So the program continues. Now there are monthly meetings for the two of you (and the rest of your family, from time to time). Professionals attend when possible, but the main feature of these meetings is the opportunity to compare notes with other couples. The areas of discussion are endless. These post-hospital meetings touch nearly everything involved in living. They offer a chance for easy, informal discussion among people who share the same basic problem and who, therefore, understand each other's problem as no "outsider" could.

The Portable Program

We have gotten ahead of ourselves—and your immediate problems—to give you an overall idea of what the Heart Wife program is, how it works, and what it does. The essence of the program is simple: women who have been through it helping women who are going through it. The best help is given face-to-face; and someday we hope there will be Heart Wife units wherever there are Heart Wives who need comfort and counsel. Until then, this book is a substitute—a portable Heart Wife program. It does what we would be doing if we had a chance to sit and talk with you: as best we can, giving you the information you need at each stage of your husband's recovery, starting with his days in the CCU and continuing.

How long? Well, we talk to women whose husbands have just been admitted to the Coronary Care Unit and to women whose husbands "recovered" from their heart attacks thirty

years ago. The "veterans" are, if anything, even more eager to
talk, even more relieved to find out they are not alone. Understandably. If your husband has just had his heart attack, you are
just discovering the problems and emotions you must deal with.
After thirty years, you know. Oh, how you know!

We know, too. After several hundred sessions with Heart
Wives of all ages, we still learn at least one new thing each time.
A new slant on how to handle a situation, perhaps one we dearly
wished we had known about when we faced that situation.

Where You Are Right Now

Let's start with the problems that are most immediate, things
you should be aware of as soon as possible.

First, you must commit yourself to facing the fact of your
husband's heart attack.

You may never find it quite "believable." He may have had a
splendid physique and an iron constitution. He may have been
a health-foods fanatic; the calmest, most beloved, secure, and
tension-free man in the world; he may have come fresh from an
EKG administered by the entire Mayo Clinic. No matter.
Everything that makes his heart attack so "unbelievable" counts
for absolutely nothing now.

He has had a heart attack.

Face it. Accept it. In fact, say it. Right now, out loud. It is
important for you to hear the actual words in your own voice. If
you have already tried to tell people close to you, you know
why. Most Heart Wives have agonizing difficulty getting the
words out at first; a good many, including one of the authors,
just could not do it that first time. Jane called her brother to tell
him, and broke down, unable to say the words she had never
heard herself say. Another Heart Wife, after ending several
attempted phone calls in incoherent tears, gave up and spent the
night writing postcards.

Get it out of your system now. Say the words out loud.

Accepting the fact of your husband's heart attack is essential, because one of the first things you must do is help your husband accept the fact of the heart attack. Unless he does, recovery is bound to be torturous and chancey. A man will not do what he must to recover from an illness he does not admit he has. And everything that makes his heart attack unbelievable for you, will likely make it the same for him. The man who "shouldn't" have had a heart attack, going by risk-profile standards, is exactly the sort of man most likely to end up ignoring his occluded arteries and, what's worse, ignoring the usual consequences of ignoring unpleasant facts. He may turn the doctor's instructions into a game of evasion, of "let's see what we can get away with without the doctor finding out." The trouble is, the doctor is not playing. He is just keeping score. And this is a game in which, sooner or later, everybody knows the score.

So, COMMIT YOURSELF TO ACCEPTING THE FACT THAT YOUR HUSBAND HAS HAD A HEART ATTACK. THEN HELP HIM ACCEPT IT.

That is the first step in surviving it—for both of you.

The Next Step

At the risk of sounding repetitious, we repeat—the next step is realizing that you *truly are not alone.* Not in your problems, not in what happens to you, not in the thoughts and emotions that sweep over you, unbidden and unwelcome. Heart Wives can help you.

Particularly during the early stages of recovery you will run into many of what we call "Checklist Problems." Most of them require nothing more than reasonably simple action on your part; but the action must be taken in time. We will help you with these by reminding you of things that need your attention. We will also help by warning you ahead of time of things you might not recognize as problems. Like the need to say the words "heart attack" aloud to yourself before trying to say them to someone else, one of the first and most common problems Heart Wives run into. It shows the value of not being alone; only those who have already been through it are apt to realize that saying "heart attack" could be any problem.

Other "Checklist Problems" are examined in Chapters 6 and 8 in the order they generally occur.

Problems of Information and Awareness

You have already seen how some of the problems affect Heart Wives. Now we will show you how Heart Wives help each other solve them.

Take the case of the Heart Wife who was so upset because she was "being closed out" of her husband's recovery by his doctor.

Other Heart Wives at the meeting immediately assured her that the same thing happened to them. That alone cheered the "closed out" Heart Wife considerably. At least she now knew she had not been a special case, marked for a special, personal put-down. She was no longer alone. Then a cardiac nurse who was at the meeting explained why such things happen to nearly all Heart Wives. Doctors invariably prefer to examine patients in private; it spares everyone's feelings and the patient has fewer qualms about being examined, about discussing his condition and answering the doctor's questions.

It is that simple. But if you are not aware of the fact, you are bound to get the notion that you, as an individual, are being "closed out" of your husband's illness because you, personally, are somehow deficient in intelligence or character, or are otherwise "unworthy" of being a part of his recovery. It is only a question of bringing the problem out into the open and giving the Heart Wife a bit of information. Suddenly, the problem disappears.

Then why didn't the doctor, himself, explain things to the anxious, hurt wife? The most sensible answer we have heard came from another Heart Wife at another meeting where the problem came up (as it often does with new Heart Wives). She said:

I don't think doctors deliberately withhold information from us. But they go through it every day. It's routine for them; it doesn't even occur to them that we don't know how they do things, or that we might want to know. Or that we could be disturbed about it.

That a Heart Wife could be upset by a common hospital routine might not occur to anyone—except another Heart Wife who has been through it, who knew what was troubling you, and who could give you the information you need.

The same is true in the case of the Heart Wife who was made to feel "like a naughty little girl" for not having "done something" about her husband's weight. At one of our weekly meetings we asked a cardiologist about the whole problem of Heart Wives who are made to feel small and incompetent by doctors, nurses, and other staff members. He asked us to remember that doctors are human, too. They have personal problems and pressures of their own that can make them preoccupied and insensitive to the feelings of people they deal with. They get tired and overwrought and testy, just like everyone else. Are you always as considerate and tactful as you might be? Well, neither are they.

While that answer may not eradicate the problem, it certainly helps if you are aware of the human factor involved.

That applies even more forcefully to your feelings of helplessness and uselessness.

Again and again new Heart Wives will bring up the subject at one of the first weekly meetings they attend. They often talk about how guilty they feel, how they are sure there should have been "something more" they could have done at the time of the attack.

If you called for help, tried to keep your husband still until it came, kept assuring him that everything was going to be all right, and smiled all you could under the distinctly unjolly circumstances, you did exactly the right thing. Anything more would have been too much. As one Heart Wife told us:

My husband had been on blood-pressure medication. And I

thought, "Well, I want to get his blood pressure down if he's having a heart attack." So I gave him a blood-pressure pill. That was a terrible mistake! They go into shock from the fear and the change to the system, and low blood pressure's one of the dangers of shock. When we got to the hospital, they said, "his blood pressure is very low," and I told them what I had done. That's when I learned about shock!

So the advice is, don't give medication indiscriminately.

Actually, the advice is, do not give medication at all! So if you did nothing, you did everything you could—and should—have done.

Once you realize you are not alone in your sense of helplessness, once you can talk about it with other Heart Wives, you quickly realize that you have been punishing yourself for no reason. The feeling of helplessness is one symptom of a large category of problems Heart Wives can help each other with simply by letting each other know they are not alone in having them. These problems come from a conflict between your identity, personality, and needs as a woman and a human being and what you strongly feel is your duty to be superhuman, totally devoted, and totally selfless. In a word, Superwoman.

We call this broad category "The Beauty Shop Problem," because one of the earliest signs of it, for many Heart Wives, involves their self-inflicted agony over whether or not to go to a beauty shop.

You naturally want to look your best (or at least not your worst) when you go into the CCU to see your husband. In fact, the doctor practically made it a prescription. He tells you to be cheerful and confident; your inner voice tells you that if your husband sees you looking the way you feel—haggard, bedraggled, red-eyed, and worried—he will assume you look that way because you think he is going to die. Well . . . the thought has crossed your mind. And you look it. The obvious answer is a quick trip to the beauty shop, maybe a rinse and set. It will certainly help physically, and we all know what it can do for morale.

Then comes the conflict. How can you even dream of going to a beauty shop now! What kind of woman, what kind of wife, could even think of how she looks with him in there, maybe dying! Who but some heartless monster would have her own looks, her own morale in mind, when . . .

But you know the rest. It is bad enough when the conflict is entirely internal, strictly between what you are (human) and what *you* think you somehow should be (superhuman). If you allow yourself to be intimidated by what you imagine other people think you should be, the conflict can last the rest of your life.

The plight of one Heart Wife we know shows how the woman-Superwoman conflict can paralyze us into giving up all claim to our own lives if we listen to any voices that speak of unremitting, selfless duty. This Heart Wife has spent thirty years since her husband's heart attack being Superwoman. She goes where he goes, lives the life he likes, does what he wants to do, with the people he likes. She has not had a vacation in all that time, but she has gone on quite a few hunting and fishing trips, to be sure he is well taken care of on *his* vacation.

The sad thing is, she never wanted to be Superwoman; she was cast in the role by her husband's strong-minded and adoring family. She has spent thirty years listening to them remind her of her husband's "condition," and why it means she must defer to his wishes entirely in the arrangement of their lives.

Whenever she found herself thinking she was entitled to some life of her own, her inner voice parroted the words she had heard for so long that they had become her own: what awful, unnatural thoughts; how monstrous even to entertain such selfish, unloving notions! Dismiss them at once, and punish yourself for having allowed them by being even more self-sacrificing, more aware of his needs.

You see? She thought she was alone. Her in-laws had convinced her that no real woman could possibly consider her own wants and needs as long as her husband had a "condition."

How can you avoid such "Beauty Shop" problems?

First, you must realize exactly what the problem is. It is definitely not whether you should or should not cater to your husband. The problem is realizing that you are not alone. You are not a singular, horrid monster for having thoughts and emotions that come to you no matter what your husband's condition. Other Heart Wives have had the same thoughts, the same emotions. In fact, most of us have. Random thoughts, even remarkably selfish ones, did not disturb you unduly before your husband's heart attack, did they? It is just that now, because of the attack, you feel you should rise above your human nature. You must be Superwoman; you must not have unseemly or selfish or frivolous or petty thoughts.

But we do. All of us. And unless you know that, you will feel singularly alone, with no outlet and relief for the strange, unsettling problems of thought and emotions you have. You would not discuss them with friends or the hospital staff, even if you figured you might get some answers, because a good part of their sting specifically comes from the way you feel sometimes like a ninny and other times like some sort of horrid, unnatural monster for having them.

You cannot talk about how you feel with the doctor, either. You know the doctor is a fearsomely busy, harried man. He may be visibly exhausted. How can you "bother" a man who is so overworked with "trivial" or "frivolous" personal questions—no matter how much they bother you? How can you take up what little time you do get with him (a Man of Science, yet!) to talk about how you feel when going to a beauty parlor? You don't get to ask him all the *medical* questions you have!

So you talk to no one. And you never discover that, far from being unique or horrid, your thoughts and emotions are absolutely routine, maybe even a little tame.

By way of proof, we offer this sampling. The Heart Wives involved had kept their thoughts bottled up, sure that only *they* were capable of thinking such things. When they found out they were not alone, the thoughts came pouring out:

I was very angry that he had this heart attack. I mean, I felt I didn't want to be a nurse. I'm being perfectly honest—I just did *not* want to be a nurse!

I tried to figure out how it would be for me if Jack died. And yet the minute I felt that way, I tried to rush it out of my mind. Because God forbid anything would happen to him with thoughts like that going on in my mind.

Suddenly I became awfully interested in what life-insurance coverage we had.

My immediate feeling was, "Well I'm going to dump you, because I'm not going to be like my mother and have an invalid, a sick old guy, around. I'm not!" I mean, I was too young! I was twenty-eight, just too young for that.

I kept thinking what I want to do is just go to bed and pull the covers over my head for about six months. I'd feel a little guilty, but it was just too goddamn bad if anyone didn't like it!

I wanted to go to the movies one night. But I was afraid that if I went to the movie, that would be the time he'd have another heart attack. Or if I went out to have a piece of pie, there I would be, stuffing myself while he's laying in the bed having a heart attack.

About two days after Pete's heart attack all I could think about was sex. I practically propositioned the doctor.

I remember going to the hospital in a low, peasant blouse with the push-up bra and the bleached-blonde flowing hair—and the whole scene.

I never had an affair with anyone. But I thought, "I have to protect myself." You know"—in case he should drop dead, I've got to have number two ready and waiting."

So, you see, you are not alone.
But where can you find that out except from other Heart Wives? As you just have.

CHAPTER

4

Save Time: Plead "Guilty"

There is this to be said for any of the other illnesses that can cause the sort of problems you are having: at least his mother cannot blame you for them. Better still, even *you* cannot blame you. But a heart attack? The second question you ask yourself—right after "Will he live?"—is, "Was I responsible for it?" And you cannot take "no" for an answer.

If I was any kind of wife, you tell yourself, I'd have watched his diet and made him take off those extra pounds. I'd have served margarine and cut out fat and eggs. I'd have made him quit smoking and cut down on liquor and take his vacation someplace where he'd really rest. I'd have kept the kids out of his hair so he could relax a little. I'd have seen that he didn't worry so much, that he didn't get so churned up over raises and promotions and how much he was making—or I was spending.

Then again, maybe you did all those things. Kept after him about his weight and overwork and never getting regular exercise and all the rest. Then what can you tell yourself? Well, what do you think gave him the heart attack? Nag, nag, nag—that's what!

Impale yourself on whichever horn of this dilemma you like; either way, you're stuck. The prosecutor (you) and the judge

(you) leave no doubt in the mind of you, the jury: the verdict is
. . . guilty.

We felt the same way; so has each Heart Wife we have
counseled. And it is not just a matter of our experience, observation, and opinion. The University of Oklahoma Medical
Center studied two groups. Former heart patients were in one;
their wives in the other. In the Canadian Medical Association's
Journal, Doctors Adsett and Bruhn noted:

> While the men dealt predominantly with the loss of self-es-
> teem, the women were concerned with guilt feelings. They
> questioned what they might have done to contribute to their
> husbands' heart attacks and felt that they were greatly responsi-
> ble as protectors of their husbands' future health.

So it is unanimous. You think you are guilty; we thought we
were guilty; the wives we see every day think they are guilty. As
for those women in the therapy group, their guilt feelings were
so pronounced, it seemed to be their main characteristic. We
cannot all be wrong.

Or can we? If you hold yourself responsible, whether you did
or did not do the things doctors say can help prevent heart
attacks, if there is no way *not* to feel guilty, then how can the
words "responsible" and "guilty" have any real meaning in this
situation?

Exactly what are you responsible for? You read in Chapter 2
what a heart attack is and what can cause it. Doctors may be
uncertain which factor was most critical in any particular case;
but at least two important factors—heredity and high blood
pressure—were clearly beyond your control. As for the other
factors—well, you could have done something about them, in
theory. But theory is not always the same as fact. His weight,
for example. If you served him an outright starvation diet at
home, you would still have no say in what he ate outside. And
even at home, short of the sort of nagging that, itself, may cause
heart attacks (and surely causes divorces), there really is not
much you can do without his cooperation.

One Heart Wife put it like this:

> Oh, I was aware of my husband's weight problem. I was
> always asking him to lose weight and to exercise. But he was
> under so much stress, with such problems, the time to live
> healthy was always in the future.
>
> I'd read an article or risk-profile and show it to him and keep
> after him to go in for a checkup, a cardiogram. "Well, I'm going
> to lose weight, first, then go in for the checkup." I'd keep at it,
> keep at it—but when a man's getting it from all sides, you don't
> want to keep nagging when he gets home. That's refuge!

You decide: Is she guilty for not having *insisted?* For not
having "kept at it" a little more? If so, how about that other big
factor in heart attacks, tension?

You can keep your home as free of tension as a Swedish
massage, but how can you keep his boss from jumping down his
throat? For that matter, how can you keep his own competitive
juices from running him ragged?

We are not saying you are not responsible and should not feel
guilty. We have no idea. But neither do you. Because you
cannot know exactly what caused the attack. Anyway, what
you think or feel about your guilt does not matter; what you do
about it is all that counts, now. And what you must actually *do* is
the same in either case. If you are guilty, you must make up for
it by doing everything you can to help him recover. And if you
are not guilty, you still want to do everything you can to help
him recover!

Of course, you can realize how complex the causes of any
heart attack are, and how little probability there is that any
single factor was the cause (least of all, casual tension between
people who, when you come down to it, love each other). You
can understand that—and still feel guilty. A Heart Wife whose
husband was about to come home told us with tight-lipped
regret that in the eight years of their marriage, she and her
husband had elevated bickering to an art form. We asked
whether she felt guilty, then, about having been a cause of the
attack.

It would have happened, anyhow. There's just too much happening with his arteries and "glycerids," or whatever they're called—things I couldn't control.

But I can help give him stress or help give him peace.

So I guess I feel sort of guilty. The thing is not to have it happen anymore between us. From my end, at least.

That is the only sensible attitude to take about your feelings of guilt, the only one that does much good.

Certainly, weeping and wailing and carrying on about how it was all your fault does no good. (If it worries him into another attack, you will really have something to feel guilty about!) Besides, it can turn into a terrible cop-out, with you washing your hands of your real responsibility—helping him recover—because you have already taken on yourself responsibility for the attack. What's more, blatant guilt feelings are likely to create a totally unnatural atmosphere for him. The two doctors at the University of Oklahoma Medical Center noted this reaction in their groups:

> Many of the wives felt very guilty about past anger, aggressive feelings, and behavior that they had expressed to their husbands, and they were therefore inhibited in expressing their feelings [to their husbands] since the husband's heart attack. One woman stated: "I had it in my head that if I said anything cross to him in any way, he could die, and I didn't want that on my mind."

You can imagine how natural, happy, and tension-free the atmosphere was in that household. She let guilt feelings turn her from a wife into an emotional tightrope-walker. And we find that same fear in too many Heart Wives.

Mousing about on emotional eggshells is not the way to avoid giving him a heart attack. "Letting off steam" when it builds up is important for anyone; for a heart patient it is vital (ask his doctor). When people who love each other get angry, letting each other know it is a sort of safety valve. And it is infinitely better than chewing over grievances, swallowing anger, choking down resentments, letting them smoke, smoulder, and churn inside until they finally erupt in an uncontrollable explosion of rage. The explosion is what's really dangerous, not the steam; rage kills, not anger.

A woman wracked with guilt over her possible contribution to her husband's coronary cannot be a natural wife. She will keep her emotions locked in, letting her resentments grow inside until the pressure is too great. Then the explosion. Her husband—who is very likely a little nervous and puzzled, anyway, as to what's come over his wife, with never a cross word or nasty look anymore—is bound to react to what will seem, when it comes, blind, unreasonable rage, out of all proportion to whatever last little straw triggered the explosion. He will strike back, tit for tat. And that could be that. All because of her guilt.

What can be done about that guilt?

In the Heart Wife program, we first point out, as we have done with you, the impossible guilt dilemma of every Heart Wife. A cardiologist explains how impenetrable the cause of any particular attack is. Then we drop the subject. The idea is to eliminate *future* guilt (where possible) and minimize it where guilt is inevitable. What's done is done; what's important is what you do tomorrow.

Unfortunately, the problems that come up specifically because of your husband's illness are in that dreadful "damned-if-you-do-and-damned-if-you-don't" category. Your choice will often be between unpleasant ways to make the best of a bad situation.

You are going to feel guilty about neglecting your children for your husband. Or about neglecting him for them. You are going to feel guilty about neglecting your household duties or other serious responsibilities. If you work, you are going to feel guilty about continuing at a time when he needs you with him. If you stop working, you are going to feel guilty about jeopardizing your family's long-range welfare.

But some choices are easy if you consider the alternatives. Maybe you feel guilty about telling relatives and friends whose visits tire your husband that they must limit their visiting time. But how will you feel about not protecting him?

In general, you are bound to feel guilty every time you have to be tough or demanding or hard-nosed, every time you do any of the pushy, brazen things your mother told you only un-popular girls do. But that guilt is nothing compared to the guilt you will feel if you do not do whatever you must to make his recovery easier—or maybe even possible.

One Heart Wife said that when her husband got home, she did not have much trouble with visitors, generally speaking. But . . .

> One person became angry when I asked her to please wait a week or so. And I felt bad. But I never felt really guilty. I knew that I wasn't doing anything wrong. I knew I wasn't abrupt with her or anything. She was just being very inconsiderate—and I had to think of him first.

Suppose it had not been a situation in which the Heart Wife was honestly able to tell herself that the other person was being unreasonable or inconsiderate. No matter. The Heart Wife might have felt a little worse about it, but she would have done the same anyway. It was a matter of setting priorities and sticking to them. First came her husband's welfare.

Doing what you have to do should eliminate, or at least minimize, guilt in most situations at any stage of his recovery (which will go on for the rest of his—hopefully—long, happy life).

You can see the basic rule even in the feelings of helplessness we discussed in Chapter 2. Guilt is the obvious result of your inability to help your husband while everyone else is helping him. And you *should* feel guilty—if it's true that you aren't helping. Because it shouldn't be a bit true! You should be playing a key role. Not only when he gets home. Not only in his long-range recovery. But now! Right in the CCU. In his im-mediate medical survival. One doctor we talked to described hospitals this way:

They're a trade-off. On the plus side, they offer fine medical care, sophisticated machines, and concentrations of well-trained people who know what to do in emergencies and who have all the equipment and medication they need, right at hand.

And it's still a trade-off.

Because on the minus side, you give up personal warmth and feelings of personal worth. You can easily feel as though you're not a person, at all—certainly not someone who's loved and needed, someone whose recovery and return home is anxiously awaited.

Instead you can feel like an object, a laboratory specimen, something that's being acted on and is strictly replaceable by any other object.

I guess the ideal would be if someone could invent a cardiac monitor that loves you.

Not that he values modern medical machines and medications less, he just values love more. And that means you. That is what you can do for your husband. And it is something the finest cardiologist, the best-trained nurse, the most lavishly equipped Coronary Care Unit cannot do. You can give him incentive to live, you can make him feel needed and necessary. And loved.

The most eloquent expression of your love will be the way you make decisions where some guilt is inescapable. If you are plainly keeping in mind his needs, it will show him how you feel about him. At the same time it will minimize your guilt when you must do something unpleasant or hurt people you do not want to hurt.

Take the problem of being with him. You can always be right there, all the time. But what if it means dropping other responsibilities—like leaving your children alone at a time that is very frightening to them, letting your house "take care of itself," maybe quitting your job? You feel guilty about taking either course. So which should it be?

Well, how does your husband feel about it? If he will be worried sick about how the children will get along with both of you away so much, he is not going to feel better and more loved because you are there, at his bedside, instead of with them. But he will feel loved and necessary if you let him know that you are making arrangements to be with him as much as possible—*without* neglecting things he wants taken care of. And he will feel absolutely essential if you talk over the problem with him, letting him know that satisfying him is uppermost in your mind.

In short, the best way to avoid guilt in deciding what's best for him is to *ask him!* He will not feel very good about your making any major, family decision without consulting him. How could you—if, indeed, you love him, need him, respect and rely on him?

There is still another reason to consult him. Look at yourself and the problems you are having from his point of view. He knows what has happened to him has scared you half to death. He knows he could die, leaving you alone. He is worried about his role as a family-provider, as a husband (both sexually and as a partner in running a family), and as a man. He has shattered your life and he knows it. Talk about guilt feelings! What you do may very well affect just how guilty he feels; how guilty he feels may very well affect how fast and completely he recovers, how he adjusts to the new life-style that faces him. Consulting him about the decisions you must make will go a long way toward soothing the anguish he feels over doing all this to you. It will let him participate in making things as right as they can be.

You can't eliminate all your guilt feelings—or his. But you can minimize them. More important, you can refuse to let them affect your ability to do the things you must do.

It is a matter, finally, of looking at all problems in the light of your real duty and responsibility—which is to do everything you can to help him recover. In that light, the choice of even the bleakest alternatives is much easier. Yes, you may feel guilty about bothering busy nurses; but you are not there to make the nurses' lives easier, you are there to help your husband. And if it means bothering a nurse or a doctor or *anyone*, that is what you must do. Obviously, we are not suggesting that you would harass the hospital staff for nothing; but if your husband needs something, don't ask—*demand.* Nicely and pleasantly, if possible; but with enough force and insistence, in any case, so that you get action.

If you base your decisions and your actions on your understanding of what your husband wants, what he needs, and what is clearly best for him, you will have nothing real to reproach yourself for.

Note the word "real." You may feel guilty no matter what you have done if things turn out badly. But if you have done your level best, all you are really feeling guilty about is the unfortunate fact that you are human and not perfect. That is "guilt" you can endure.

CHAPTER

5

What Are They Doing to My Husband?

The fact that your husband has had a heart attack is frightening. The fact that he needs to be in a special unit setup for twenty-four-hour emergency treatment is frightening. The strange-looking, Space Age Gothic machines are frightening. The needles plunged into his arm are frightening. The sight of anyone having to breathe with an oxygen mask is frightening. And the monitor! That is the most frightening of all! The pulsating blip on the oscilloscope, the jagged, sawtooth pattern showing his heart beat; the dials, the cold electronic numbers —and that ominous little red bulb with the word "alarm" over it. Alarm? Panic is more like it.

One Heart Wife's reaction the first time she saw her husband in the CCU sums it up:

> I didn't realize what was going to happen ahead of time. What I'd be seeing. I didn't stop to think; I just went right in.
> It was the scariest thing I ever saw.
> I looked at him, then I looked around and saw other patients,

and some looked like—well, suddenly I couldn't stand it. I just ran out of there, tears falling out of my eyes.

It's very frightening!

Very frightening. For anyone. The sight of someone you love in a CCU is such trauma that any reaction you have is perfectly understandable. Of course, the odds are you will not run out of the Unit. But if you do, it will most likely be in order to get a policeman to come and put a stop to what looks an awful lot like an updated Spanish Inquisition.

You know the CCU is necessary. But that does not do a thing for your fright. It will always be frightening to a woman whose husband is in it. But it can be less frightening if you know what you are looking at, what the various machines and instruments are, what they are used for and why, and how they will help your husband if needed. So let's take a close look at a CCU.

We recently took the closest possible look, guided by Dr. M. C. Thorner, a cardiologist who teaches at USC Medical School, is Consulting Cardiologist for the Los Angeles Police and Fire Departments, and still finds time for private practice as an attending physician at the Cedars-Sinai Medical Center. He took us through the cardiac floor of Cedars of Lebanon Hospital. It was a coronary show-and-tell, with Dr. Thorner pointing out everything you are liable to see and wonder about when you go to your husband's bedside; he explained what everything is, what it does, and how it helps heart patients.

He started with the equipment. Most of it is for one of two purposes: to give the earliest possible warning of arrhythmias or to correct them before they can do any damage. The basic reason for a CCU is to give the heart time to heal itself, to keep the patient free from strain, work, emotional stresses, and ten-sion-building pain.

But that is not what it looks like to a casual observer. And to a wife, whose observation of the scene is anything but casual, what is happening to her husband may seem calculated more to create stress, strain, and pain, than to diminish them.

That needle sticking in his arm, for instance. *That's* conducive to stress-free, painless rest?

Well, no. But neither is it causing any discomfort. What you see is an intravenous injection (IV), a simple precaution our guide explained this way:

Dr. Thorner: The intravenous solution is going constantly.
H.W.C. (Heart Wife Counselor): So it does not mean—
Dr. Thorner: It's routine.
H.W.C.: It isn't because anything's wrong?
Dr. Thorner: No—that's explained to all patients when they come in. They get an intravenous that runs all the time, just in case they need emergency medication. That's all.

He went on to explain that the colorless liquid you see in the container the needle and tubing are attached to is a glucose or sugar solution. If your husband suddenly needs medication, there will be no time lost finding a vein, no fumbling around inserting needles. The doctor or nurse simply injects whatever drug is needed into the IV tubing or substitutes a container of necessary medication; either way, it is almost immediately at work in your husband's blood system.

The IV will stay in as long as your husband is in the CCU, or in the Coronary Observation Unit. In fact, a sight to cheer the heart (of wives, anyway) is a patient who is near release taking exercise his doctor has ordered by walking the corridors, pushing along what looks like an old-fashioned, upright hatrack on wheels. Hanging from the tip of the shaft is an IV container; a tube hangs down and disappears up the patient's bathrobe sleeve.

After the IV, the next most prominent sight in a CCU is one most Heart Wives find even more disturbing—once they know what it is. Long after you have gotten used to the sight and idea of the IV, you can still spend a lot of time nervously eyeing the cardiac monitor screen.

The frightening thing about monitors is that you can actually *see* what is wrong with your husband's heart. Or—you think you can, anyway.

It is truly ironic how monitors, which are probably the biggest single factor in the gratifying decline in coronary deaths, are also the greatest source of misapplied fretting and worrying for Heart Wives!

A cardiac monitor is to an electrocardiogram what a fluoroscope is to an X-ray: it is not as precise or complete; but it is *now*. Electrodes are taped to the patient when he arrives: on his chest, lower abdomen, sometimes arms and legs. But instead of recording the heartbeat on a strip of graph paper, the monitor shows the beat on an oscilloscope screen (although, when needed, the tracing can also be made on a graph strip). The monitor does not have to be as precise as an EKG; it is for warning, not diagnosis. And it is peerless at its job. It shows exactly how the patient's heart is performing at that exact second. The doctor and nurse do not even have to be watching. At the first sign of irregular rhythms, the monitor sounds a piercing electronic beep and a red light flashes on. It is highly noticeable.

Before monitors, doctors and nurses had to hope the patient would notice any irregularity of beat, or give some sign, or that someone would catch it on examination. Now the monitor tells everyone, out loud and unmistakably, that something is wrong; and the monitor does it sooner than the best cardiologist could if his stethoscope were glued to the patient's chest every second.

Does that sound ideal? It is—for everyone except Heart Wives. The trouble is, the monitor speaks only one language: electronic-display-on-an-oscilloscope-screen. Which is Greek to most of us. Here is what Dr. Thorner said about your chances of correctly interpreting what you see on your husband's monitor. He was showing us a nurses' station for an Observation Unit; it had a bank of monitor screens.

DR. THORNER: Here you have four patients being monitored at the same time. If anything happens to any one of them, a red light goes on and there's a noise.

Quite often there will be alarms because the patient has moved suddenly. Then the nurse looks at the monitor, and if she sees there's nothing wrong, she just clicks it off.

H.W.C.: One of the wives we talked to was very disturbed because that line on her husband's monitor was jumping all over the place.

DR. THORNER: When you're dealing with electronic equipment, things can happen to it. A patient can even knock an electrode loose, and it's going to go completely off.

Every alarm doesn't mean that a patient's in trouble. *Most* don't.

H.W.C.: Would someone with no training in reading the monitor be able to tell what it means about the patient's condition?

DR. THORNER: No, they'd have no way of knowing. Patients will be doing this on the monitor . . . [*he points to a particularly jagged tracing on the screen*] and they'll get real disturbed about what they see; and I'll say, "Well, you're just moving around, that's all."

The patients have no way of knowing. Oh, after they've been here a while they get to recognize what's going on. Some of it.

H.W.C.: How about a wife coming to see her husband?

DR. THORNER: Someone coming in that seldom wouldn't know; she wouldn't see it enough to know the difference. No. That's part of the price you pay for being in a sophisticated Unit.

All things considered, it is a pretty small price to pay. Especially now that you know there is no reason for your alarm at what you *think* you see—or even, most often, at what you hear when an alarm sounds. The monitors, after all, are only machines, however sophisticated; they are designed and set to sound off whenever anything is "wrong." But, to them, the irregularity of heart rhythm because of sudden movement, strenuous stretching, or a loose electrode is . . . wrong. And they say so, with a hair-trigger response. That is what makes them nonpareils when it comes to warnings of arrhythmias. A cardiac nurse can glance at the screen and tell in a second why the alarm sounded; on the other hand, it took her a good number of years to become a cardiac nurse. You cannot successfully rush the process; you cannot learn in the course of a few visits what the tracings mean. And you will save yourself considerable grief if you do not even try.

If you possibly can, just ignore the monitors.

You can't? Well, that is scarcely surprising; they are designed and placed so they cannot be ignored. But at least keep in mind the reality of the situation. Unless you have had training in cardiology, the tracings on the monitor are guaranteed not to mean what you think they do about your husband's condition. *Guaranteed!* If you think your husband is doing well, the tracings will seem such a jagged, ragged mess (which they are), you will be sure something is wrong. And if your husband is having a hard time of it? The tracings will still seem hopefully symmetrical, with regular repetitions of pattern (which they are). The fact is, the appearance of the line to our untutored eyes has no particular relationship to a patient's condition. What's more, there is no valid comparison you can make between your husband's monitor and that of any other patient. Your husband's "blip" may be higher or lower, more or less ragged-looking, with peaks spaced closer or farther apart than another patient's. All that means is that they have different hearts, different kinds of attacks, with damage on different parts of the heart; in short, they are different people. It does not mean that one is sicker than the other.

So much for amateur monitor readings.

Much of the other equipment you will see all around him will be in the same place and same condition all the time—untouched and unused. Those things are for emergencies. Two exceptions (besides the IV) are the main monitor, right over his bed, and a blood-pressure machine (sphygmomanometer). The main monitor is bigger than those at the nurses' station and more elaborate. It will probably have a dial to show pulse rate, plus some electronic wire-numbers (the kind that glow on electronic adding machines) for blood pressure. These may not be working. That has nothing to do, good or bad, with your husband's condition. Those readings are not as accurate as ones taken by hand; unless there is some reason for a running rough estimate of pulse and blood pressure, they are not used.

The hand that takes pulse and blood pressure belongs to the nurse. If your visit is interrupted by the nurse using the blood-pressure cuff, it does not mean anything is wrong, except, perhaps, that she has been so busy, her schedule is a trifle off.

In addition to the blood-pressure machine on the wall behind your husband's bed, you will see a number of electrical outlets, plus some curious-looking valves. These are for oxygen supply and for suction.

There will also be a strange kind of clock. It has a minute hand and a second hand, but no hour hand. Furthermore, it is divided into minutes, but has no hour markings. And it is not running. Hopefully it will not be. It goes along with the two other major pieces of emergency equipment standing nearby. They are a positive-breathing apparatus and a defibrillator.

The positive-breathing apparatus is a waist-high pole on a stand. It ends in a sort of knob on which there are some controls. Sprouting out of the knob are what look like two rabbit-ear antennae, but a little thicker, not tapered, and rigid, rather than telescoping. These can be attached to an ordinary oxygen mask or to a variety of tracheal tubes that are introduced down a patient's throat. The apparatus breathes for the patient, filling his lungs when they are not operating. It is part of cardiopulmonary resuscitation (the pulmonary part, to be exact) and can help bring a patient back to normal breathing after incidents that would have meant sure death not many years back.

The defibrillator (the premier "cardio" part of "cardiopulmonary") is a rectangular box some two feet long, a foot or so wide, and less than a foot deep, about the size of an overnight bag. On its face are a couple of simple dials. Leading from its base are two flexible cables; they look like rubber accordion hoses, one black and the other red, each ending in what looks like a single stereo headphone. You have probably seen a defibrillator in simulated use on one of the TV hospital shows. The two electrodes (those headphone things) are put on the patient's chest, the switch is thrown and the defibrillator gives enough of an electric shock to disrupt a dangerous arrhythmia and get a patient's heart back to a normal beat. Or, if the heart has stopped, to shock it back into action.

These machines are not needed in most cases. The more tractable arrhythmias can be handled by various drugs, perhaps in combination with closed-chest massage. When massage is needed, another item you will see at your husband's bed goes into action. That is a bedboard, which looks like nothing but a three-foot square cutting board in your kitchen. And that is about all it is: a board slipped under a patient, so the person giving the heart massage will have something harder to push against than the mattress.

In any emergency, that strange clock behind your husband's bed comes into its own. It is a giant stopwatch. It is started when treatment begins so the resuscitation team can tell exactly how long any treatment has been administered, whether it is time to try a different treatment, and how long it will be until any drugs they have given will start taking effect.

The drugs they may use will come from the "Crash Cart."

Depending on how many beds are in the CCU, you will see one or more Crash Carts. They look like busboy's carts, stainless steel, about four feet long, three feet wide, and waist-high, with a push bar at one end. There will be a defibrillator on its top, along with various containers of medications, and a good many more drugs, swabs, syringes, tubes, and other hospital impedimenta in the trays that fit into the cart's open-sided body. Each Crash Cart is a complete, mobile, cardiopulmonary resuscitation unit. And there is at least one on each floor of the hospital. The entire medical and instrument repertoire of the cardiac-arrest team is there. Furthermore, every member of a modern hospital staff is trained in cardiopulmonary techniques.

Naturally, you will also see many of the things you could expect in any doctor's office: stethoscopes, thermometers, and the like. Plus a few things that will look familiar enough so that you will barely notice them, although they are actually specialized CCU items. Automatic rotating cuffs, for instance. They are tourniquets used to restrict the flow of blood coming from the arms and legs, so that a reduced supply of blood returns to his heart, giving it less work to do.

Except for the IVs and the oxygen masks, though, the chances are you will not see any of the specialized equipment in use. It is used; in fact, your husband is very likely to see some of it in operation, although with the less dramatic instruments and with any of the medications he probably will not be aware that anything noteworthy is happening, perhaps not even if he is the patient!

Any time an emergency procedure is necessary, you will be asked to leave. The curtains are drawn and the staff gets to work. Not that they have anything to hide, or that what they are doing to the patient is too horrid to view. It is to cut down on any attendant excitement for the other patients and to keep them from being disturbed by the activity. It is also out of consideration for the patient being worked on, and for your feelings. Two ways. First, you would certainly feel awful if you happened to get in the way during an emergency (though not quite so awful as the family of the patient whose emergency treatment you interrupted!); second, you have emergency procedures near enough the forefront of your mind, as it is, without being there to see one.

How about your husband? Will he find it disturbing?

Not really. For one thing, he is quite sedated, as part of the no-stress, no-strain kind of resting his heart needs. More important, the chances are excellent that the procedures he sees will be successful ones. And it is a reassuring sight for a heart patient to see the speed, efficiency, and elaborate care given by a cardiac team.

What *will* you see going on when you visit your husband? As little as possible. Remember that the purpose of the CCU is to keep a patient's heart beating—slowly, evenly, and with as little work to do as possible. As we said, that is one reason he is sedated (the other is to make sure he has no pain, a fairly essential condition for rest). For the same reason, he is prodded, poked, palpated, and generally fussed over as little as possible, since none of those is much conducive to rest, let alone sleep. However, "as little as possible," in a CCU, is not all that little. You will see nurses giving medication, taking pulses and blood pressure; you may see them talking to patients. It is not idle chatter. One sign that is important in a CCU patient is how the patient is feeling. And the patient is still the best "machine" for that particular reading.

There is one more thing you may see; and we would like to say a word about it. You may see a bed, now empty, that had a patient in it the hour before.

Remember this: CCUs have cut the mortality rate in half. Advances are still being made. In fact, Dr. Thorner showed us a research machine—one of only five in the country—that may make deep inroads on the number of deaths caused by two conditions that are much more refractory than fibrillation (though, mercifully, much, *much* more rare). If so, if the new counter-pulse machine can help keep victims of cardiac shock and cardiac failure alive long enough for healing to begin, the mortality rate will go down farther.

It will never reach zero.

The important thing for you to remember is that the moment your husband entered the CCU, his chances shot upward. And they are improving every minute, now.

CHAPTER
6

Decisions, Decisions . . .
(A Slightly Expanded
Checklist)

This may be the only time in your life when you are well-advised to put off making decisions. As many as you can. Probably until your husband is out of the Coronary Care Unit and settled in a regular room; certainly until you are out of shock and settled into enough of a routine so that you have time and concentration enough to weigh decisions with the care they deserve.

Not that your judgment is necessarily bad, even in shock. But we all tend to feel committed to decisions we have already made. And everything is so hectic for you right now, chances are that many decisions would be dictated by circumstance, rather than actually *made*. You are improvising, taking things as they come. So you do well to consider most provisions you must make—about the hospital, doctors, your home and family—as temporary expedients. Firm decisions about most of them can wait for a while.

Some decisions, though, cannot wait. You must make them immediately. They may not be more important than others you can safely put off. But, like weeds, they quickly get out of hand if not tended to. Cope with them now and they are nothing; let them go and they can become elaborate and burdensome problems.

They are the "Checklist Problems" we mentioned earlier. This chapter is a checklist to remind you of some things that must be decided—and an expanded checklist where discussion is necessary to warn you of other things you might not realize *need* decision. No one is more urgent than another. But they do generally come up for Heart Wives in the order we present them.

Ready? Start checking:

Who Should Be Told?

The answer is not automatically "everybody," or automatically "nobody." Or *automatically* anything. It is definitely a decision to be made. And the only sensible answer is, "It all depends."

List everyone you might tell. Then ask yourself the same questions about each: Is there any reason so-and-so should *not* know, at least right now? What possible *bad* consequences could there be? Who could be hurt—and how? The person who is told? My husband? My family? Me?

Start with parents, brothers and sisters, particularly close relatives, and dear friends.

One Heart Wife decided not to tell her husband's mother for the simplest of reasons: she was afraid it would kill her.

The older woman had suffered several heart attacks herself and was bed-ridden much of the time. But even that sort of decision is not automatic. First, the Heart Wife had to weigh the chance of her mother-in-law finding out about the heart attack in other ways.

> You know, the grapevine. I didn't want it to filter back to her. I didn't want her to learn about it in a shocking way. It'd be even worse than if it came from me or his brother.

First of all, I wanted to get him over the hump. Then she would be told with the proper people in attendance—her doctor, and so on.

Medical reasons for not telling most often apply to parents. It is more of a shock for them and they are most apt to be of an age, or in a state of infirmity, where extreme shocks can be dangerous. But it is something to keep in mind before telling anyone. If there is the slightest question, play safe and consult the person's doctor before telling.

We must add that some Heart Wives disagree. They feel that, this side of almost medically certain disaster, not telling anyone who has a keen, personal interest in your husband is wrong. The most impressive argument for that viewpoint came from a Heart Wife who said:

> I think you have to tell people, even if you're afraid how it may affect them. Because if something happens, they've got to know ahead of time, so it isn't such a terrific shock—so the first thing they hear won't be, you know, "Well, it's all over." *What's* over!

There is something to be said for that. But we still think there definitely *is* a decision to be made, if only because of the possible chain-reaction shock, the news of your husband's heart attack killing or prostrating someone close. How will *that* news affect *him?* Or wouldn't you tell him? In which case, why not *start* not telling at the beginning? Where it does the most good—or, anyway, the least harm?

At any rate, right or wrong, that kind of decision is reasonably easy to reach emotionally. You are thinking of *them;* if you withhold the information, it is in their own interests. The next sort of decision is much harder because it is based on a wish to spare yourself, not the other person. It may appear to be an intensely selfish act; it is bound to crush and infuriate the person not told.

A Heart Wife who lives in New York was faced with just this sort of decision. Her widowed mother, who lives in the

Midwest, was on the first leg of a month-long group cruise. She was flying to New York, and the plan had been that the Heart Wife and her husband would meet mother at Kennedy Airport, spend the evening visiting, then take her to the steamer for a midnight sailing. The heart attack happened the night before. And as the Heart Wife told us,

> I decided my mother couldn't be told.
> First of all, it would ruin her trip. But, mostly, it was because if she canceled and stayed on, I wouldn't have been able to function. You can't hold yourself together when you're trying to hold everyone else together.

She met her mother as planned, explaining that her husband had been called out of town on business. She took her out for a long dinner and delivered her to the ship, then dashed back to the hospital. The only indication that her mother thought anything was wrong was when "I kept 'excusing myself' and running off to the ladies' room; that's where the phone was! Mother finally said maybe I ought to see a doctor because didn't I know that was the first sign of diabetes!"

Another Heart Wife was even more explicit about her reasons for not telling. Her husband's mother is an excitable, nervous woman with an advanced talent for setting everyone on edge. And her son led the list of people who got very nervous when she was around. Fortunately, she lived on the opposite coast.

> I had a quick talk with the doctor, and we decided that it would be better if she didn't come.
> As his mother she had a right to know. But, then the most important thing was for my husband to get well. And for me to *stay* well, to help make him well.
> Having his mother there would have been difficult for him —and impossible for me. I simply would not have been able to handle it. She would have gone to pieces, and it just would have brought me down.

Whether you are trying to spare the person or spare your

husband and yourself, you must take into account how you can plausibly hope to keep the information from reaching the person. In these three cases accidental discovery was not much of an issue. But all three Heart Wives realized that their decisions required some action to implement them. As yours will. If only to make sure everyone who does know and who might be speaking to the other person understands that there must be no mention of the heart attack.

Of course you know what can happen to even the best-laid plans of mice, men, *and* Heart Wives. The news may leak out despite your most thoughtful precautions. Furthermore, the people you do not tell now are bound to find out sooner or later; in fact, if all goes according to plan, you will probably be the one to tell them. And you must realize that when they do find out—no matter how or from whom—you are in for some pretty intense resentment and recrimination.

The most soothing answers we have found to the inevitable hurt and outraged "Why wasn't I told?" are (1) a reasonable facsimile of the truth: you decided to wait until it was clear that he was out of danger, since there was no reason they should have to worry when there was nothing they could do to help. . . , or, (2) a perfectly plausible, face-saving lie: you waited, because no one was sure it was a heart attack until just now.

There is one more possibility to consider. You may conclude that you stand no chance at all of keeping the news from some people whose presence at the hospital is a clear threat to your husband's recovery (or your sanity). There is only one course of action that offers a faint glimmer of success: lay it on the line; tell them you know how emotional and easily upset they are—and this is not a time when you can allow your husband, or yourself, to have any upsetting influences. You love them, and hate hurting them—but *that's it!* Said with enough gentleness and sincerity, such things need not cause irreparable damage to the relationship between you. Maybe. In any case, first things first. And first comes your husband's survival—and yours.

CHILDREN

Actually there are three groups of children to consider. Infants, youngsters, and young adults. Those too young to realize what is going on and who need maximum care, those old enough to understand, and those old enough to do something about it (like help with the first two groups, for instance). Roughly speaking, the dividing line comes at four or five between toddlers and youngsters, and anywhere from twelve to fifteen for young adults.

With older toddlers, the question is what to tell them and when. They know their father is not home. Where is he? For that matter, where are you much of the time? And why? "Daddy's sick" is no answer at all. They know what "sick" is; they have been sick themselves, and they did not go away. Far from it, they specifically had to stay home. Qualifying "sick"—like "very, very" or, "sick in a grown-up's way" will not help much; it leads to more questions. And before long they start asking breath-taker number one, "Is daddy going to die?" That is going to cause something of a pause in the conversation. You will not be prepared, even if we prime you with answers other Heart Wives have given (once they got their breath back, that is), from a lighthearted, "Why, of course not, darling!" to a grim, "Not if I can help it!" There is no all-purpose, "right" answer. The one you come up with, on the spot, will be the best.

As a guideline, though, remember that the truth, while lacking the stunning clarity and absolute simplicity younger children prefer, requires fewer supplementary answers, a lot less time, and nowhere near as much ingenuity—important points, since you do not figure to be at the top of your form, right now, what with the strain and all.

Besides, you have to tell them about a heart attack eventually, if only to explain their father's condition when he comes home and to prepare them for the restrictions and dislocations it will cause around the house. So the only real question is when to tell them. The answer to that is—as soon as possible; as soon as you have the patience and concentration necessary to explain what a heart attack is and why they can't see him now.

With youngsters from about age five or up, you probably have no choice. You know your children, of course, and we do not. But if they are five or over, we bet you stand next to no chance of getting away with any shilly-shally about what is wrong with their father—not even long enough to give you a breathing spell while he is still in the CCU. Besides, in almost every other area the only safe assumption to make is that your children know more about any given subject, atomic physics to sex, than you think they do. So, as a kind of reward for honesty, it may be that they can explain heart attacks to *you*.

Certainly, many Heart Wives have been delighted at the maturity of their youngsters' reaction. One floored us with . . .

Mrs. R: While I called the rescue squad, I had my son get on the other phone to call our doctor, who happens to be a close friend of ours, and . . .

H.W.C.: Your son is how old?

Mrs. R: Seven.

H.W.C.: So a seven-year-old called the doctor?

Mrs. R: Oh, yes! I said, "I want you to call Uncle Jerry and tell him Mommy says Daddy is having a heart attack and to come immediately."

Well, he called and the service answered. So he made them track Jerry down. I mean, it's amazing what children are capable of!

But of course, he *is* a little boy. So, naturally, the next thing he had to do was call in the whole neighborhood . . . [*laughing*] to come and watch the ambulance!

One caution: no matter what you finally decide to tell the children, by all means tell their favorite teacher or the principal of their school. If they are not yet in school, make sure whoever is with them knows. That is equally important whether your

children know or not. If they do know, they may be acting a
little strangely, and some responsible adult should be aware of
why. If your children do not know, a teacher will find it a lot
easier to handle things the way you want them handled if he or
she knows what the situation is. And, face it: in an emergency a
lot of time and explanation will be saved.

Naturally, you will tell any young adults who are living at
home. Especially since you will be counting on them, from the
age of twelve or so, on up, to be a main source of help with
everything (including any younger children) and senior
partners in your own, domestic Mutual Aid and Comfort
Society. The sooner they know, the sooner they can start
helping.

With adult children who are living away from home (or
children of a previous marriage) there is some question of when
they should be told and who should do the telling. One Heart
Wife covered both considerations that might persuade you not
to tell adult children right away. She has two adult sons and a
daughter, all of them married, all living in different cities. She
decided to put off telling them until her husband was out of the
CCU,

> . . . to spare them the hell I was going through for the next few
> days.
>   Also, I didn't want them to come trooping in to see him—and
> I knew they'd come, no matter what I said. He'd have thought it
> was the Last Rites, or something.

How important is it to forestall dramatic, long-distance visits
by people who will feel they *must* come and see your husband,
no matter what you say? Here is an answer from a patient who
had undergone by-pass surgery following a heart attack:

> There's nothing like waking up and seeing all those faces
> around the bed. There's your father and your mother and sister
> and your sister-in-law and your son! He's so busy studying, he
> can't even take time to write letters home. But there he is! All

those faces, turned down at you: "Did I die, or what? What're they all *doing?*"

Oh, there's nothing like it!

It surely is a point to keep in mind.

Other points to consider are who should tell them if they are not your children, and, in some cases how to tell them.

Just the fact that they may be his children, not yours, does not necessarily mean you should not be the one to tell them. It depends on your relations with them. And on their age. If they are quite young, you do not have the right to make the decision—certainly not until you have talked to their mother —and to your husband.

How younger children are told is important when they happen to be away from home. One Heart Wife's twelve-year-old son and eight-year-old daughter were at a summer camp when their father had a heart attack. Instead of phoning, she waited one day then went to the camp to tell her children in person and to assure them the doctors said their father was going to be just fine! Her face-to-face message had important results, because she planned to leave them at camp.

> I decided it was better for them to enjoy the summer and be with their friends, not stay around home, worrying every time I left the house.
>
> It worked out fine! And the vital thing was going to tell them in person. They could look at me and see that I wasn't devastated, that I was telling them the truth when I said their father was going to be all right.

His Employer, Business Associates, Customers, etc.

Is there any reason people connected with your husband's work (or your work—or both) should not know about the heart attack?

— Will his livelihood automatically be affected if his employer or associates know he has had a heart attack?

— Will he lose a chance of promotion or be shifted to a dead-end job?

— If he is in a profession or is self-employed, will his clients or customers abandon him for fear that a man with a heart attack can no longer serve them?

If your answer is yes, you should obviously keep the news from as many business associates as you can—everyone if possible. More likely, though, you will not be able to decide either way. So why not wait and see? Certainly until you have had a chance to talk it over with your husband. Do not rush to tell any business associate who does not absolutely have to know. You can always tell people tomorrow; but you cannot make them forget tomorrow what you told them today.

The same goes for people you work with. Could you lose your job or chance for advancement because of your husband's heart attack? Are the people you work for likely to fear that you will be too busy taking care of your husband to take care of their affairs? If so, honesty may not be the best policy; it may not even be a sensible one. Especially since it will certainly be a lot easier to keep the news from your employer or clients or customers than from his.

However, it may not be possible to keep it from his associates. There is simply no chance if:

— Your husband is covered by group insurance through his company (whether the company pays all, or part, or none of the premium);

— As company policy, someone will have to verify his illness;

— His work regularly involves heavy physical labor or some hazard that will be impossible for him to return to;

— His superiors or coworkers are solicitous enough to visit him, but are "company men" before they are friends, and will undoubtedly report back (even their suspicions, if not allowed to visit);

— Until your husband returns to work, your family income will include State Disability or Workmen's Compensation.

Under any of those circumstances, your husband's employer is bound to find out exactly what has happened. But the consequences may be much less gloomy than you think. While some changes in your husband's work situation are nearly inevitable, they are not necessarily for the worse. (We will examine the reasons, and ways he can turn the heart attack to advantage, in Chapter 11.) By all odds, the least likely consequences are out-of-hand dismissal or demotion by an employer or mass desertion by clients.

On the other hand, if you treat a heart attack as something to be kept secret—and you are discovered—everyone is apt to accept your evaluation. "Why would they try to hide it unless he was really in a bad way? Maybe we better start looking for a replacement." That sort of thing.

Still, we repeat: there is no need to rush. Do not tell anyone who does not *have* to know, and maybe not even them until you have had a chance to think over the possible consequences, and can discuss them and the "need-to-know" list with your husband.

FRIENDS, RELATIVES, AND ACQUAINTANCES

From your point of view, "need to know" is also the criterion for deciding which friends, relatives, and acquaintances to tell and which not to tell. But with two substantial differences. The only "need" to consult is yours, not theirs. And it is not a matter of keeping the news from anyone, just of not having the news come from you. At least for now.

It comes down to this: whom do you feel you need? Maybe in the waiting room, between visits to the CCU. Maybe at home. Who do you think can best be of specific help, if you need any, caring for your children, shopping, cooking, traveling, and so forth? The people to tell are those you expect will be a help to you, whether by their actions or just by being with you. And those are the only people you should tell right now.

Your choice should have nothing to do with closeness of

relationship, either by blood or friendship or even affection
under normal circumstances. That is why we include acquaintances. A number of Heart Wives have mentioned that at this
critical period they found themselves turning to people they
considered strong and reliant, even if they were not especially
close friends, rather than to much closer friends whom they
prized (and still do) for other, less stalwart qualities. Right now
you need helping hands; and even the closest and dearest cannot
help with hands they are constantly wringing.

That is from your point of view. Your husband may have a
different list. Ask him if there is anyone he particularly wants to
have know about the heart attack—or not to know. The first is
much more important because of the cards and notes notifica-
tion will evoke. In fact, if there is any conflict—if he wants you
to be sure and tell good old Harry, when the last person you
want to see right now is Mrs. Harry—you can answer the
inevitable "Is there anything we can do" with a grateful "Keep
those cards and letters coming," forestalling offers of com-
panionship for yourself with any polite lie that springs to mind.

Visiting

How much time will you spend at the hospital while your
husband is in the Coronary Care Unit? And later, when he is in
a regular room? The second decision is, of course, only tentative, but you should try to make both now because other
necessary decisions and arrangements depend on your answer,
as you will see.

There are three parts to both decisions. You must figure out
how much time you *want* to spend at the hospital, how much
time you *can* spend, and how much you *should* spend. Let's look
at them in order.

How Much Time Do You WANT to Spend at the Hospital?

You may want to be there every possible minute; then again, you may not. Either is "right"—if it is truly what you want, not just what you think you are supposed to want or, worse, what you think other people expect you to want. Here is where many Heart Wives run into a particularly nasty form of "The Beauty Shop Problem," the conflict between the real woman you are and the Superwoman you somehow think you should be, impervious to human wants, having no emotional needs of your own in the face of your husband's need.

Remember, much of any time you spend will literally be *at the hospital*, not with your husband. Certainly, while he is in the CCU, you will spend fifty-five minutes in the waiting room for every five you spend with him. And even later, unless he is in a private room, you may have to do a lot of waiting between visiting hours. For some Heart Wives, that does not matter; it is very important to them to be there, whether or not they are actually with their husbands. They often feel it is equally important to their husbands. As one Heart Wife put it:

> I know he felt better just knowing I was on the other side of the door. And it was where I wanted to be, even if I didn't actually get to see him any more often.

Other Heart Wives find the endless wait unbearably taxing. One who felt that way told us:

> I asked the doctor if he thought I should stay here, and he said, "No." I said, "I'd rather be at work." And he said, "I quite agree; you do not belong in the hospital—you'd be a basket case." I said, "Yes, I would."

Fine. In both cases. The thing is to be clear in your own mind just what it is you truly do want.

However, knowing how much time you want to be at the hospital is not the end of it.

HOW MUCH TIME CAN YOU SPEND AT THE HOSPITAL?

Your time may not be entirely your own, which means that the decision may not be entirely up to you.

First of all, there may be specific commitments that necessarily keep you from the hospital. And even if you can ignore some of them, doing so may not be a good idea from the standpoint of helping your husband. He is there to rest; you are there to help him rest. And you will not bring him the peace of mind and heart's ease that is conducive to rest if you are at the hospital when he feels you should be somewhere else. Such as? Home, taking care of the children, if no other arrangement seems satisfactory. Or at work, if your salary is vital to your family's finances. Or wherever. The question is how uneasy he will be at the notion of your sitting outside the CCU, rather than tending to something he feels is more vital than the five fleeting minutes each hour you can be with him if he is awake (an improbable assumption, given today's repertoire of sedation).

List all the places you might be instead of the hospital. For any reason. Now ask yourself about each place: how important is it, realistically, to be there rather than at the hospital? How important does he think it is? Where would he prefer you to be?

Then CONSULT HIM.

That is a key point. See how he feels about priorities. In addition to helping you make up your own mind about how much time you *can* spend at the hospital, it will be another vivid reminder to him that you are deeply concerned about his wishes and his best interests, about helping him rest easy.

You may wonder why this decision is a two-step process. Why not simply find out what he wants you to do, then do it? Because the world has not suddenly shrunk to the dimensions of a Coronary Care Unit, and time is not measured exclusively in fifty-five- and five-minute segments. There is another aspect to deciding how much time you spend at the hospital, now and later.

How Much Time SHOULD You Spend at the Hospital?

You must make up your own mind, basing your decision on a clear-eyed appreciation of what your job is—helping your husband rest—but without losing sight of everyone's long-range best interest. His, the rest of your family's, yours. Which means your answer may not be the same as his. But if you have reflected, giving his wishes their full, grave weight, then doing what you think best is really just a slightly oblique approach to his long-range best interests, too. For instance . . .

You should not be at the hospital when you know there are essential things you must do—even if he does not agree.

Many years afterward, one Heart Wife we know still becomes visibly angry describing the wrenching demands on her time that her husband made, at what she felt was the expense of her children's welfare:

> He *insisted* I be there every hour—every *minute*. And that was *it!* I could do whatever I wanted with the kids—but I had better be there.
> Well, I figured, my kids were little and they could survive it.

Maybe so. But could she? For that matter, *should* she? She felt terrible about having given in to his unreasonable demands. And was she really helping him? It poisoned their relationship; she told us she was terrible company for him. From time to time we all demand things we should not have.

You should not be at the hospital when, for whatever reason, your presence disturbs him.

A Heart Wife who was at the hospital every day told us she "sat there and tried to make conversation and tried to be pleasant." Her husband's "conversation" consisted mostly of attacks on her as a poor cook, bad mother, and terrible wife. Dumbfounded and crushed, she "couldn't fight back for fear of giving him another heart attack." But even sitting there seemed to enrage her husband. Her solution? She went to the hospital later and later each day.

Should she have gone at all?

Not if she was going to take into account the purpose of her visits: to help him *rest easy*.

You know yourself; you know him. You know how the two of you get along in various circumstances. You will surely know when, for whatever reason, your presence is disturbing. If so, your answer should be "No." Strangely enough, you should give the same answer for the opposite reason, too.

You should not be at the hospital when your presence has too good an effect on your husband!

Strange, but true. It is not all right if he becomes too emotional or too excited or too stimulated at your visits. As one Heart Wife told us:

> When I went in to see him, his heart started going real fast—and they were going to make me leave.
> I leaned over and said "Calm down—or I can't stay." And after that, I would not stay more than a few minutes each day. That was the hardest thing in the world—to go and see him for five or ten minutes and then leave!

Hard—but best. And necessary.

If the heart monitor goes "tilt" every time you enter the CCU, the cardiac nurse will take steps. She may even appeal to the doctor to have your visiting restricted (and, of course, you should be totally cooperative).

It often seems odd to new Heart Wives that they are not supposed to do *everything* they can to pep up their husbands.

At one of our weekly in-hospital meetings, a Heart Wife was agonizing over her inability to jolly her husband out of his gloomy depression. The psychiatric social worker who was at the meeting pointed out that some depression is neither remarkable nor unexpected (it does not take a chronic worrywart to be kind of down, lying in a CCU following a heart attack). What's more, she went on to say, moderate depression is not altogether bad! It does tend to keep him quiet, low-key, and relaxed. Which is exactly what the doctor wants. So it might be a mistake for you to incite your husband to manic cheer (plus being the neatest trick of the year, if you somehow managed it). Of course, it is unlikely you will.

It takes considerable cheering to bring him *up* to mere moderate depression. The psychiatric social worker was simply telling the Heart Wife not to fret about an inability to chase the clouds away and make her husband all radiant smiles, that it would not necessarily be good even if it were possible. She was not saying not to *try*.

As our psychiatrist friend said earlier, a heart monitor can save his life, but it cannot make him feel loved or feel like living. That is your job. Which means . . .

You should not be at the hospital when you are unable to do your job.

There is no point in going to see your husband when you yourself are too sick, too tired, too choked-up, or too dispirited to do anything but drag down his spirits.

Or when you look that way.

You may be prey to any number of the inner conflicts we call "Beauty Shop Problems," but there is absolutely no question about whether or not you should *go* to a beauty shop. You should do anything that makes you look, feel, and act better, more confident, and more cheerful than—well, than you feel. And you should not go near your husband until you have done whatever is necessary to get yourself looking that way.

One Heart Wife, who, keep in mind, is a truly stunning woman, said it this way:

> It rests with us. We can help our husbands live by making them know we want them to live.
>
> Or we can kill them—just by not seeming to care, not even looking like we care.
>
> Anytime I really don't feel like fixing up, like pulling myself together, getting my hair done, I remember how important it is to my husband that I continue to look good and feel well—which

kind of go hand in hand. If I don't do that, he's going to see right
through me, and it's going to bring him down.

Because he cares—he cares that much about me! And he sees
I care! I've watched wives come in looking like such . . . *frumps!*
No wonder the guy doesn't get well! This old . . . *thing* walks in.
She doesn't look like she cares or seems to care, so how in the
world is she going to make him care?

I mean, these wives had to bring their husbands back. And
they came in looking worse than their husbands did!

As she said, it rests with us. Maybe not, always, whether our
husbands live or die. But certainly how they *rest*.

To make sure your husband rests easy, start by deciding how
much time you WANT, CAN, and SHOULD spend at the
hospital.

Children

The scope and elaboration of the arrangements you must make
for the children depend on how much difference you think there
will be in the amount of time you were home—from the
children's point of view—before the attack, and how much you
will be there while your husband is in the hospital. For all your
children know, you make daily trips to the moon while they are
in school or routinely anywhere else away from home. So if you
decide to limit your hospital visiting to those hours when your
children are routinely away from home, there is no need to
make any particular arrangements. But since that would mean
no regular visiting, nights or weekends, realistically you will
have to make some provisions for their care. It is a good idea to
make them now, for the entire time, rather than as you go along.
This is a time of severe and mounting disruption in your
children's lives, with more than enough inherent insecurity and
drama; they do not need the added uncertainty of not knowing,
day-to-day, who will be taking care of them tomorrow. The
free-substitution platoon system may be fine for football; when

applied to "substitute Mommies," it can make children feel
disconcertingly like footballs themselves.

One Heart Wife who had left her two-year-old with a suc-
cession of sitters while she was at the hospital said:

> Finally, the baby . . . he actually refused to have sitters. I
> know he's only two—I don't have to listen to him—but he
> became so . . . *horribly* . . . *upset* at the thought of a sitter! He'd
> say, "I'll stay myself." It was his way of saying he was sick of
> Daddy being sick.

She had to adjust her decisions about the amount of time she
could spend with her husband; her children's welfare meant she
should spend less time than she *wanted* to. And her husband
totally agreed. It shows how interrelated these decisions
are—and why you should make the basic ones we are discussing
as early as possible!

So, who should take care of your children when you are not
there?

The short answer is: whoever is most fond of the children
(and vice versa) and will be most regularly available.

Usually that means relatives. The most likely are, literally,
the closest—brothers or sisters who are young adults. It is a good
arrangement all around. The young adults can feel they are
helping; the infants and youngsters can feel a little less strange
about their living arrangements. It must not be at the expense of
the older children's own sense of security or their well-being,
though. They must feel comfortable with the responsibility.

Next down the list are the children's grandparents, their
aunts or uncles, or other close relatives. But we mean close in
affection and familiarity, not just blood. A friend of the family
who has always known and loved the children is more suitable
than a relative who either has barely met them or for whom they
feel no affection.

It may seem that we have overlooked an obvious solution—
sending the children off somewhere. They could stay with a
nearby relative or friend if school is a problem, or you could
send them to a camp or almost anywhere if it is summer or they

do not go to school. After all, it is just until their father gets home. Why, it might be a treat for them!

Maybe so, but we have yet to meet a Heart Wife who, having done that, would do it again. And it makes no difference how much of a treat the trip would be under normal circumstances. For instance, Jane's mother-in-law lived in Philadelphia. She doted on her grandchildren. They, in turn, adored "Mussy." Each summer, one of her "California grandchildren" went to visit, and came back with such glowing tales, the next in line would nearly die waiting for *his* summer to come. The summer of Arthur's heart attack happened to be David's turn. With some uncertainty (on both parts) Jane sent him off. Had there been a Heart Wife program then, she would have known better. Certainly, he had a nice time (the mind boggles at what "Mussy" and "Poppa Andrew" probably arranged to distract him!); but just as certainly he did feel "shuttled off" and "sent away, out of the way." And so would your children.

Look, it's their *father!* He is terribly ill; they are frightfully worried about him, you, and themselves, and there is not a thing they can do to help. They cannot even go see him. They are just in the way. They know it, and they hate it. What's more, you know exactly how they feel; it is exactly the way you felt in the hospital corridors those first few hours, and maybe still do. In the way. Helpless. Shunted aside and left out. Now suppose someone had the authority to send you away. (And if you imagine the CCU staff wouldn't if they could, you had better lie down and rest for a while.) They would not have to send you very far. Just next door, say, where someone would "take care of you" and where you would be out from under foot so the medical staff could get on with its business, having one less problem to worry about. How would that affect your basic feelings of helplessness and being in the way?

So much for sending the children somewhere.

The problem of whom to bring in becomes less troublesome the less you plan to be at the hospital. If you decide your visits will be mostly during the day and not constant, perhaps you can count on friends or neighbors. One Heart Wife came up with a most interesting and valuable variation: "sitter-playmates." If she knew she would be at the hospital when her children would be home from kindergarten, she arranged with neighbors to have a slightly older child—maybe a lordly third-grader—be at the house. The neighbors were delighted to help and took obvious pains to select those of their children they thought would make the best, most conscientious "sitters."

With one essential thought firmly in mind, you cannot be far off, no matter whom you choose. You are arranging to have your children cared for. Not just supervised, cooked-for, told yes, they have to do their homework, and no, they can't stay up to watch *The Late Show. Cared for.* It may include all those things and more; but it also must include *caring*.

The younger the children, the more critical the arrangements. But any children who are living at home, even if they are working or in college, rely on their parents for a good part of their physical needs. Ignoring the fact can create resentments that are totally unnecessary because they are so easily avoided. A five-minute chat on ways and means while their father is in the hospital will show that you are still thinking about them and their needs. You probably won't have to make any actual arrangements; the young adults, from the age of twelve or thereabouts, can take care of their own meals, plans, transportation, and the rest. They will simply feel better knowing that you have considered the problems and are making a special effort to be sure their lives are as little dislocated as possible.

Your evident concern is crucial here. They do not feel a bit less worried, helpless, or in the way than their little brothers and sisters. Giving them a chance to assure you that you "mustn't worry about them," is a considerable service. Particularly for younger teen-agers. They seem to be the ones who are most profoundly disturbed by their father's illness. They do not yet have an adult's experience with life's changes and uncertainties, but they are old enough to have a keen awareness of how serious the situation is and what it could mean for the future. They also have the capacity to vividly fantasize unimaginable possibilities of changes in their lives.

Whatever you decide, whatever arrangements you make, there are two concerned parties to consult before any plans are final: the children and their father. The younger the children, the more important it is to be sure they are comfortable with the person who will stand in for you part of the time. For obvious reasons.

And it may be even more important that your husband feel comfortable about who is taking care of his children while he "monopolizes" your time.

Right now he is feeling pretty low about the effects of his heart attack on you and the children. Recent events have brought human mortality forcibly to his mind, and most men feel quite strongly about their children. Their personal immortality, if you like. So what you do to insure that your absence (on his account) has an irreducible minimum of bad effects on your children at a most stressful and worrisome time in their lives—those arrangements are bound to be of towering interest and concern to your husband. And, as in all other such areas, just the fact that you show concern for his concern will mean a lot to him.

Logistics

The logistics of living are sort of the stage directions of our lives. They are not dramatic, not even very important; they take very little concentration or attention to get through. But ignore them and everyone on the scene stumbles about.

Your home has never "run itself" before; it won't now. This checklist will help you consider what arrangements should be made to keep things running smoothly.

CLEANING

If the sight of dust annoys and depresses you, it is sensible to make sure none is around. You do not need peripheral annoyances at this point in your life. On the other hand, if you were always relatively relaxed about housecleaning, you will not become overly excited about it now.

In either case, if you are going to spend long hours at the hospital, you are not going to feel much like cleaning when you get home. So, no matter what your standards, you can probably use some help. Here are some suggestions.

Are there children old enough to help? Can you afford hired help? Have friends or friendly neighbors offered their services? Relatives (his or yours)?

Gardening

The exact same list of helpers can be used. And the same considerations of whether you need help.

Pets

Who will care for them, feed, water, and walk them? Is it better to think about boarding them out?

Shopping

This is something your young adults, even older youngsters, can help with. If none of your children is old enough, neighbors can shop for you on their own trips to the market (and they will be glad of a chance to help). But you should prepare a list for either children or helpful neighbors. "Anything at all," is the only shopping instruction that really is any trouble; then someone has to guess what you really need.

Cooking

Again, young adults can handle it. But if you have none, make sure that whoever does the cooking when you are late or not there at all knows about the children's "pet hates." Favorites are not as important; chances are that will come out. But few people think to ask, "What don't you want?" This is going to be a time of enough turmoil for the children without meals being a hassle for want of a simple list.

Transportation

If a car is a necessity and you have no car or do not drive, check with the hospital social-services department to find if they have any suitable suggestions. If your husband is in a teaching hospital, one connected with a medical school, there is probably an Office of Student Employment where you may find a driver for a lot less than a cab costs.

Or how about a car-pool system among the other Heart Wives? That way you can start your own "Counseling Group."

Insurance

Medical costs are not outrageous. They used to be outrageous, ten or fifteen years ago; now they are simply impossible. Literally. Unless you are very rich or very poor, you flat-out cannot afford any major illness today. If you are poor enough to qualify, you can get excellent, if often somewhat impersonal, medical attention, free. If you're rich enough . . . well, after the illness is over, you will be notably less rich.

For the overwhelming majority of us in between, insurance is an absolute necessity. Mercifully, many men are covered by a company group plan. Or they have their own hospital insurance with such organizations as Blue Shield. However, coverages vary widely, and a man may have more than one policy, including some of the more sporting kind advertised mostly on cards that fall out of your Sunday newspaper. They charge outlandish premiums but offer handsome cash payments when you are in the hospital, regardless of other coverage.

You should know exactly what coverage you have and how much is allowed for which services. It is a nasty shock to find out when the bill comes that some kind soul, solicitous of your husband's comfort, has put him in a private room, although your insurance allows no more than the semiprivate or ward rate. The same applies to special-duty nurses. If he needs something that is not covered—well, you will manage. But even in those cases, hospitals will very often cooperate, breaking up their charges in ways that take advantage of what your insurance does allow. But you must make such arrangements immediately. It is too late once a charge has been submitted and turned down; even the most tolerant of insurance companies will give you only one try.

It is no secret to hospitals that they will probably be paid by an insurance company. So they are fairly knowledgeable in the field. And most have someone who can answer your questions about insurance. The same is true for your doctor. Someone in his office is practically a specialist in insurance and in protecting your rights to maximum coverage (which, after all, may involve his rights to be paid; fair enough, surely!).

But in both cases, you will have to ask; and you will need a copy of the insurance policy (or policies) in hand. The best-informed expert cannot explain the ins and outs of an insurance policy that is not there.

If there is any trouble about payment by the insurance companies, if you think that you have been treated unfairly—even after you have complained and been given an explanation of their actions—you have one powerful recourse before it gets to be a question of lawyers. Just repeat the magic words: "I'm going to write to the State Insurance Commission." Letters going to the state commission cause enough bother so that insurance companies would rather settle any close dispute in your favor.

THE HOSPITAL

CHAPTER

7

Doesn't He Want to Live?

It is awfully ironic. Suspiciously like a bad joke. You have been assuring your husband, assuring your children, your family, and friends, telling them all, over and over, "Everything's going to be . . . *all right!*" And now, just when you get the first demonstrable sign that it actually *is* going to be all right after all, you run smack into a possible danger point.

Your husband is ready to leave the Coronary Care Unit!

Depending on the setup and sophistication of your hospital, he may be going to a coronary observation room. That is sort of a CCU without tears: even if there is a heart monitor, it is better-safe-than-sorry insurance, not something to be watched with such steadfast anxiety as its cousin in the CCU. Or your husband may go to a regular room. Perhaps even to a different floor. And there is nothing like the physical evidence of his moving out of the grim, hand-wringing tension of the CCU to make the point to you. He is getting better. No, he *is* better!

Naturally, you are delighted.

And your husband? He is, in part, nervous, irritable, and depressed.

He probably will not show it openly. And that is where the danger lies. In your happy relief, you may not notice how he feels. And the clash between his feelings and yours can surely damage your relationship. What can you do about it? Do not let the clash occur.

There is no clearer instance than this of how a Heart Wife who has been through it can arm a Heart Wife who is going through it with vital information. Because all it takes on your part is awareness of the problem. With that, and a few precautions, poof! The danger evaporates! First, we have to talk about your feelings. When we say your husband's reaction to the first joyous news you have heard since the attack may be something less than ecstatic, you naturally are amazed. Almost hurt. Shouldn't he welcome the news that he is now well enough to leave a place specifically conceived and appointed for constant watch against the arrhythmias and arrests that can kill him? Shouldn't he rejoice that the immediate emergency is officially over? Doesn't he want to live?

Yes. As a matter of fact, he does. But his apprehension is not a question of fact—certainly not the physical fact of his condition. It is a matter of emotion and his perception of security. Remember, your view of the Coronary Care Unit is apt to be vastly different from his. You can marvel at the machines, at the skilled personnel and their miraculous, life-saving techniques. But it is still the place where your husband could have died. You sat outside, cringing every time a monitor alarm sounded. You started in fear whenever a nurse seemed to be moving a fraction faster than usual, because speed suggests some emergency. The CCU saves heart patients' lives, but sitting outside can just about kill wives!

His point of view is different. In every sense, he has been living with those marvelous machines. Some he has been hooked up to, the rest are right at hand, ready to go to work in an instant. During the fifty-five minutes of each hour you spend outside, wondering, he is inside. And he does not have to wonder; he knows he is all right. A monitor alarm might startle you; but he knows that particular bell is not tolling for him. As we explained in Chapter 5, it may not be for anyone. If it is, your husband gets an inspiring demonstration of what the word "efficiency" means: the cardiopulmonary resuscitation team at work. He has sixty seconds every minute, twenty-four hours every day, of the best care in the hospital.

And now they are going to unplug him!

No heart monitor. No specialists practically hovering over him night and day. An emergency response has to take longer where he is going, even if it is right next door. He is leaving his electronic womb. How can you expect him not to be apprehensive? Certainly, he is also bound to be as elated as you are that the doctor feels he is progressing. The trouble is, the elation is evident, the anxiety is much harder to notice.

An article in the *New England Journal of Medicine* calls it, with unusual charm, "weaning anxiety." In the study reported, twelve of forty-five patients admitted to the researchers that they were quite anxious about being "unplugged"—just over 25 percent of the patients studied. Does that mean the chances are three to one your husband will not have weaning anxieties? It depends on whom you are talking to, on what you say, and what you listen to. The researchers asked the patients how they felt about leaving the CCU and listened to the answers; if a man said no and did not otherwise let on he was anxious, no it was. Under those rules it is surprising even a quarter of the patients said they were nervous about leaving the security of the CCU—that they were, in effect, "chicken."

Andrea Frazier is a cardiac nurse who acts as liaison with patients and families for a leading team of heart surgeons. She never asks patients whether they are nervous about leaving the surgical version of a CCU. She assumes they are!

> Of course, I don't keep count, but I'd say that nine out of ten men will ask how far away from the CCU will they be, and do the floor nurses have cardiac training. They don't make a fuss. I mean, it's no big deal, the way they ask. But they want to know! They're—"nervous."

We are convinced that virtually every man will experience at least a twinge of anxiety at leaving the security of a CCU. And we are equally convinced that very few men will admit it, except by the sort of oblique questioning Andrea Frazier regularly encounters. There are three reasons. First, this sort of apprehension has a peculiarly "unmanly" quality about it. How many men would ever say, "Hey! I'm afraid to leave home?" Well, in this case, "home" is where the heart monitor is. Second, he does not want to appear ungrateful for being alive, and certainly not ungrateful to the doctor, whose judgment your husband's apprehensions might seem to question. Finally, he sees how thrilled you are and does not want you or the children to feel let down, either by his doubts or by him, if he should die. Apprehensive or not, he *wants* to believe the doctor is right; he just may not want to be surrounded by such unrestrained joy in the face of those quiet apprehensions.

The possibilities for tension between the two of you in this situation are clear. Your unrestrained joy at his move from "that place" just has to grate on the secret, dark part of the spirit where unreasonable and unreasoning fear lives in everyone. To him you may seem callous and unfeeling, unconcerned with his real best interests, blithely disregarding the nagging worry he will not tell you about but does not realize you are not aware of.

Except, now you are aware. And that takes care of any accidental clash between your attitude and his.

Now. What can you do about the substance of his apprehensions—his nervousness over leaving the security of the CCU?

This is one problem you decidedly should *not* discuss with him. That would only be rubbing in something that he is embarrassed about—not one of the better ways to ease tension. And there really is nothing to discuss. Just some simple things to do. You start with some powerful allies: the objective reasons for your unmixed (and his only slightly adulterated) joy. Make the most of them. Or, better still, ask the doctor or nurse to. Have them stress the fact that patients leave a CCU only when there is no longer any reasonable need for constant monitoring (which is somehow more reassuring than the usual announcement to a patient that he is "ready" or "is coming along well enough" to leave; patients do not want promotion—they want security).

Maybe your husband will be moving to a coronary observation room. Or to a room on the same floor as the CCU. The similarity of one or the closeness of the other is also worth stressing.

Whatever the location, your husband's new room will unquestionably be a lot more comfortable, cheerful, and, above all, more private (any place, including the proverbial Macy's window at high noon, is more private than a CCU!). Not that he will be lonely in any sense. Medically speaking, he is still a heart patient. The nursing staff knows it and is aware that he must have more—and more prompt—attention than most other patients. He will also be able to have visitors. And he will have you there more than five minutes an hour.

A patient either needs a CCU or he doesn't. The crucial part of an emergency (*anywhere* in the hospital, but right in the CCU is equally far away) is spotting it and calling for help. A minute's difference before the appropriate therapy begins is not the end-all or be-all. So your husband will not be released from the CCU until the doctor is positive he is past the stage at which there is going to be the kind of sudden, no-warning arrhythmia that must be detected almost before it begins and dealt with *now*. If your husband has any problems, they will develop much more leisurely at this point. And the floor nurses will respond in plenty of time.

You might also set up a little demonstration of how attentive the nurses are where he's going. Explain to the charge nurse what you are doing and why. Then, at the first plausible opportunity, ring for something—water, an aspirin for your headache, anything—and have a nurse primed to pop right in. Don't make it a question of "I told you so," though. If you must comment, make it in the form of a "confession." Tell your husband you were the tiniest bit—not worried, exactly—concerned about how comprehensive the coverage is in the new location. And how relieved you are to see it's so quick.

If, despite all, it seems from his remarks to you or to the CCU nurses (ask them) that he is concerned about being left alone, take advantage of relaxed visiting hours. The first day arrange to be with him almost constantly, perhaps being spelled by an appropriate relative. Or arrange for special-duty nursing the first twenty-four hours.

As the ultimate guideline, just keep in mind that the object is to spare your husband the necessity of either feeling anxious *or* owning up to his anxiety and having to ask for reassurance. But there is nothing wrong with your seeming anxious is there? If you think you can carry it off convincingly, you can be the one, right from the start, who has some slight apprehension. You can appear to be the victim of "modified rapture" at the news that he is leaving the CCU. You can ask the cardiac nurse and the doctor for reassurance, doing the asking when and where your husband can hear. You do not even have to rehearse anyone; the answers you will get are exactly the ones you want.

Your husband may even supply some of them! Because nothing will calm his fears faster than helping explain to you why they are groundless.

And nothing will demonstrate to him so dramatically your concern for him. You do have to be convincing about it. But that should not be hard: you are concerned!

CHAPTER

8

The Handwriting on the

Ceiling

You have probably used the phrase "the handwriting on the wall." Certainly, you know what it means. When people see the handwriting on the wall, they know the party is over.

The handwriting your husband sees may be on the ceiling, because he spends so much time flat on his back, staring up. But the message is the same, wall or ceiling; as a modern version of this granddaddy of all graffiti might put it, "You've had it, buddy."

Has he?

He cannot help but wonder, given his state of mind at this point. And you must understand what that is, or his various attitudes will be incomprehensible. He may deny that he has had a heart attack and blithely do things in defiance of the doctor's orders—and common sense—that seem calculated to give *you* a heart attack. He may undergo a personality change that makes him seem totally different from the man you know, love, and married. Worst of all, he may become hostile toward . . . *you!* For no reason, with no warning.

Actually, we have never spoken to a Heart Wife whose husband did not have at least one of those reactions; and it is by no means unusual for a man to have all three. That is how we can know what is going on in your husband's mind. Now . . . why should these things happen?

It starts with shock.

"What happened?" the victim of any major trauma asks. "What hit me?" It may have been a two-ton truck—or a heart attack. There is the same stunned, disoriented confusion. So, right from the start, your husband was not thinking any too clearly. And his first thoughts were none too comforting.

While he was in the CCU, his mind was a jumble of questions. The big one, of course, was will he live? But by the time the doctor could practically guarantee the answer is "yes," further questions were just as troublesome. What kind of life will it be? What will he have to give up? Smoking? Drinking? The foods he likes? Sports? Activities? Social life? Suddenly he is faced with the possibility of a life without zest or flavor. And those are only the little pleasures!

How about sex? What will the heart attack mean to that part of his life?

How about work? Whatever his ambitions, his goals, plans, and dreams, they will now seem to be ashes. How can a man who has had a heart attack expect to compete?

What gives this whole line of thought its damaging power is an uncomfortably rich larding of truth. He is not imagining the problems. He *will* have to give up some things, cut down on others. His life will change.

Sex is definitely out for a while, and he knows it. But how long is a while? Forever? One patient—who is also a doctor— told us:

> The total effect of a heart attack is a terrible sense of emasculation. You lie there and you're aware of how weak and impotent you feel—and, maybe for the first time since puberty, you know you have no sexual drive, no interest even.
>
> And I don't mean just specifically sex. I mean you don't feel like a man—it's just disappeared. All vital, masculine feeling. It's just gone. You're defeated. And you don't see how it can ever come back.

As for work, his concern can range from worries about career advancement to how he will support his family. There *is* a certain prejudice against men who have had heart attacks. At a meeting of ex-patients, one said they were looked upon as sort of "taboo." Another said that big corporations are often told by insurance companies to avoid hiring men with heart conditions or promoting them too high, otherwise group insurance rates would soar. Is that true? It is easy to suppose an employer will be leery of allowing a recent heart-attack patient to command a position of such responsibility that, if he should have another attack, the organization must falter. What can your husband do to allay such fears? Promise never to have another heart attack?

This threat to your husband's career can be even more demoralizing than the moratorium on sex. The doctor can convincingly assure him his enforced continence is temporary. A man's work is different. No one can *assure* him of anything. Even before the heart attack your husband could not be sure he would achieve whatever his goals are. Now he may convince himself that he is washed up.

Think what that does to him!

Most people want to be winners; we say that we are a nation of winners and we admire winners. Men may talk about what a "rat race" they are in, earning a living, getting ahead. But they seem to try awfully hard to run well in that race—"cardiac personalities" more than most.

Now, suddenly, your husband fears he may be disqualified from the race, not even allowed a chance to compete, let alone win. Obviously, that means he cannot be a winner. He will be a loser!

It is bad enough that he will be counted a loser in the eyes of "the world"; how about what he thinks he sees in your eyes? Your disappointment and, perhaps, scorn? What has he done to *you!* One Heart Wife said that when she was allowed into the CCU for the first time, she was amazed to find that her husband's dominant mood was desolate self-reproach:

"He just felt so bad! He said, 'You got a dirty deal.' "

Think about that. "Dirty deal" implies more than rough luck or a bad break; it says you have been cheated. You entered into what used to be called the marriage contract, and the other party to the contract "did you dirt." But cheating is conscious, as though the heart attack were intentional. Silly? Not entirely. Even if you never said a word to your husband about his physical condition, he probably has been telling himself for years that he really should take better care of his health. He didn't. And now look! He is bound to feel some measure of guilt over his own self-neglect. And that will be a good measure of how much guilt he feels about what he has "done" to you.

Let's sum up your husband's probable state of mind.

He has had a tremendous physical and mental shock. His thinking may be made even fuzzier (necessarily) by sedation. He has spent days brooding over his dim prospects. He knows he must certainly give up many pleasures. He will not be able to function, sexually, for many weeks, perhaps months. He may find himself counted out of the "race" that he always saw as an important measure of being a man. Finally, he has disappointed and let down his wife and family.

In short, he feels to one degree or another impotent, helpless, useless, and guilty.

At this point, every patient we have ever talked with or heard about asks the same questions. Why me? What did I do to deserve this? Why not someone else? (Names furnished on request.) The answer is right there, before his eyes; it is the handwriting on the ceiling. He has been weighed in the balances and has been found wanting.

The next step in this gloomy chain of "reasoning" is practically automatic.

Since the handwriting on the ceiling tells him that all good things have gone out of his life because of the heart attack, the obvious solution is not to have a heart attack! Deny it. Ignore it. Maybe it will go away. If not, at least his constant, anxious awareness of it will. That is his only defense against what he sees as an awful future.

The impulse to deny any severe sickness is evidently a commonplace, almost expected phenomenon. The same doctor/patient we quoted earlier told us:

> I was amazed at my own reaction. I see denial in patients all the time; it's one of the things I know I must always be on the lookout for in my patients.
> And, suddenly, there I am, denying to myself that I've "really had a heart attack." I knew what I was doing and how silly it was, but I couldn't help myself!

If a doctor who knows exactly what denial is, how it starts and how it progresses cannot help telling himself he has not *really* had a heart attack, is it any wonder most other patients do the same? Of course, like the heart attack, itself, your husband's denial may be of any intensity and severity. Here is one Heart Wife's description of about as strong a denial as we have run across:

> The doctor told me it was definitely a heart attack. But my husband wouldn't accept it. And nobody had told me, then, that many men don't accept the fact that they've had a heart attack.
> I finally spoke to a girlfriend whose father had heart attacks when we were in junior high. She said, "You know, to this day my father insists he's never had a heart attack." Well, he's been in the hospital I don't know how many times. I can't believe he doesn't think *any* of those were heart attacks!
> Anyway, the doctor said to my husband, "You've had a heart attack." The cardiograms showed it. But two minutes after the doctor walked out he was telling me it wasn't and I should tell friends it wasn't. Which left me in the air. What do I tell people? He's in intensive care with . . . *nothing?* It left me really crazy!

Not many men carry denial that far. But we suspect most men deny their heart attacks to some extent, because the result of denial is almost always the same: the patient does things the doctor has particularly forbidden. And that happens so often, even with men who do not deny the fact of their attack out loud, that a special-duty nurse told us she hates taking male cardiac cases:

> It's too frustrating! They won't follow orders, they won't admit they've even had a heart attack. "What does the doctor know?" They'll show him; nobody's gonna tell them.
> Then it starts—seeing how much they can "get away with."
> *Bedpan? Them?*
> You turn your back one second, and they're halfway to the john.
> Hurrah! They fooled the dumb nurse again!

Chances are they do not even fool themselves. So why do they do it? Time and again, we find Heart Wives distraught because their husbands seem bent on a suicidal disregard of the doctor's orders. One called us in tears; she had just come from her husband's room, where she found that some (alleged) friends had brought him a carton of cigarettes, which were now neatly tucked away under his mattress. We started to explain about denial. But she said, "He knows he had a heart attack; he doesn't deny it." Not in words maybe; but he is showing that he does not fully accept it. Of course, he is not going to get up and walk out of the hospital (which would be true denial); after all, he felt that pain, he feels the weakness. Instead he compromises by flouting particular rules he sees as only the overcautious part of a heart patient's regimen.

Shuffling to the bathroom rather than using the bedpan; sneaking the odd smoke.

In effect, what he is denying is not so much the heart attack—just what he assumes must be aftermath. Is it bad or dangerous for a heart patient to smoke? His reply is, "Well, then, heart patients certainly shouldn't; and I must not *really* be one because look, I'm smoking!" Not pack after pack, maybe, but you can get a lot of defiance and denial out of a simple, cautious drag. *Especially* in a hospital.

What can you do about it?

Show him that the *real* delusion is that message he thinks he

sees written on the ceiling: he has not been "found wanting."
The future, while certainly different, is not necessarily bleak.
Your life together will be different in the future. But it has been
different in the past! Your separate lives changed when you got
married. That life changed when you had babies. It changes, in
some degree, with every promotion or job change; it changes
dramatically if you move from one city to another. This is
another change. What makes it seem so different is that it is not
voluntary. But in a number of ways, this change may be *less*
comprehensive than many of the previous major changes. And
the detailed changes in diet, habit, and life-style will probably be
a distinct change for the better.

You see, now, the reason for our admittedly fanatical insistence on saying over and over CONSULT HIM about
decisions. The most important single message you can get
across to him is that YOU WANT HIM TO GET WELL; it
will continue to be the message. Clear through this book, clear
through your life together.

Will that do the trick?

Of course not. When was life that neat and simple?

The shock and apprehension of a heart attack is too great to
be dispelled by a few minutes or hours or days or months of the
most earnest reassurance.

He will probably have some temporary personality change.
He will probably be hostile toward you for a while. And that is
during the relatively short time he is in the hospital. He is likely
to become hostile again, in a different way and for different
reasons, when he gets home. Remember this: BOTH BOUTS
OF HOSTILITY AND PERSONALITY CHANGE *ARE*
TEMPORARY.

The personality change in the hospital can be so dramatic it
will probably frighten you, even though we have told you about
it. (But imagine what it is like when you do not know how
expected, normal, and temporary it is!) A few Heart Wives
have told us they were so unsettled at the time that they found
themselves thinking that if he was going to be like this the rest of

his life, well, maybe it would be better if he . . . didn't survive. Yes, it can be that scary. It generally seems to be in reaction to whatever the man fears most about the effects of his heart attack. If anyone tells us that is much too pat and simplified, pop psychology at its cocktail-party worst, we will give in immediately; we really are not very sure. It does not much matter. Nor does it particularly matter why these personality changes are temporary. They happen; they end.

Given the rich variety of human behavior, we cannot begin to tell you exactly what your husband's personality change will be like. But it may console you to hear about a few of the more extreme changes Heart Wives have mentioned. Just so you will know the worst that can happen. Very often they are either overtly sexual, or at least involve an assertiveness that suggests a man reassuring himself about his masculinity.

That is so generally the rule, we think of these as a whole category of problems you can expect to face—"The Grand Turk Problem." Most women find it harder to seek help for this kind of problem than for the problems of actual sexual adjustment that come along later in recovery, once their husbands are home. The "Grand Turk" is so wildly unexpected, so "abnormal"—no matter how permissive your notion of what constitutes "normal" in sexual attitudes—it may seem somehow disloyal to your husband to discuss his behavior with anyone; surely not with anyone who even possibly might not understand.

For example, although Mrs. B's husband was not at Cedars-Sinai, her sister knew about Heart Wives and called us to explain that Mr. B had had a heart attack about five weeks earlier and that, for the past two weeks, Mrs. B had seemed more and more distraught. All she would tell her sister was that "Something is wrong with Harry." Not physically wrong; he was coming along just fine and would be going home in a week or so. Would we call Mrs. B and see if we could help?

The phone call lasted a little over an hour and a half. It seemed that Mr. B, who was in his early forties, was normally a very dignified, quiet, and considerate person. Now he had suddenly turned into a dirty old man! There he was, in the hospital, leering at nurses, patting, pinching, reeling off dirty jokes, broken only by suggestive remarks. At one point the Bs' teen-age daughter left the room in tears and shock.

We told Mrs. B that personality changes like her husband's (though, admittedly, not always quite so marked or bizarre) are almost the rule with heart patients. We told her about other cases, how they had been just as unsettling for the man's family. And, more important, how each had run its course in a matter of weeks. We quoted one Heart Wife whose husband had taken to the most outrageous language and had been giving a pretty passable imitation of the Grand Turk, flirting with every woman who entered his hospital room or who walked by his open door. "Three weeks later, at home, he couldn't believe he had acted like that. Really! He thought I was making it up, to tease him!"

Mrs. B calmed down considerably.

Her sister, on the other hand, got pretty excited. In fact, flabbergasted. She assured us, later, when Mr. B. was back home, stoutly denying he had ever said any such things, that her sister was not the sort of woman who discusses her husband's mild idiosyncrasies with strangers, let alone such behavior! It was amazing!

Not to us. Mrs. B *had* to talk to someone about it. Remember, she did not know her husband's behavior was not abnormal. She could not tell anyone about it, but we did not have to be told. We knew—and could tell *her!* The "Grand Turk" can be any heart patient, no matter what he is really like.

For instance, here are the notes we made immediately after visiting Mr. L at the insistence of his wife:

> Mr. L is a very mild-looking man. He has a pale, childlike look about him, and he never spoke above a whisper. . . .
> Mrs. L said he was unable to feed himself or walk. . . .

The floor nurses had a somewhat different view of Mr. L.

Especially the time they saw him running down a hospital corridor, totally nude, screaming that the nurses were attacking him.

Another Heart Wife told us:

> My husband changed. His personality changed, and he was . . . wild!
>
> He's usually so nice to everybody, and he won't complain. But he was ordering everybody around and complaining all the time he was in the hospital. I kept saying, "This isn't like him."
>
> And he wrote letters to the Assistant Everybody in the hospital complaining about the service, and he had me go down and Xerox them.
>
> And then he'd have me move everything around in the room and I had to fix the bed just so. Once, three women he works with came to visit, and he had them change the room all around again.
>
> It frightened me—because he rejected me. Twice I went away crying because he'd been so mean. "Fix my bed this way—NOT that way. THIS way!"
>
> He had never talked to me like that!

That personality change lasted as long as any we have heard about. Around two months, ending a week or so after he came home from the hospital.

The first indication you have of a personality change will probably be your husband's unaccountable hostility toward you. As one Heart Wife put it:

> When I told some friends Bill was acting like a maniac, they said, "Do you think he's taking his heart attack out on you?" Which I had never thought of. It just isn't his nature! He's always been so kind, so considerate of my feelings, it never would occur to me. He'd take his heart attack out on . . . *me???*

Good question. Why, of all people, *you?*

One Heart Wife was so disturbed by the question, she took it to a psychotherapist she had gone to for treatment some years before. He explained, she told us, "that hostility of this sort is not at all uncommon and that these resentments [against God or

Fate or chance or heredity or saturated fats or demanding, conniving business associates—whatever he decides is to blame for the attack] had to be directed toward someone stronger than himself."

Maybe. We were not struck by an overwhelming aura of strength about this Heart Wife, while her husband did seem to have quite a strong personality. But we would scarcely argue with a professional (as much through prudence as humility; who knows when they may start burning heretics again?). We would add the fact that a Heart Wife is the most handy target for her husband's hostility. You are there; most other people are not. You are familiar; others around him are not—and most of us are polite to strangers, even if we do not feel very well. Besides, no one can go on raging against Fate (or even cholesterol) forever. Sooner or later you want a more pliable, more satisfying target for your rage. That, classically, is how cats get kicked. Also wives. And since cats are not allowed into hospitals you are "it."

You may even end up playing a sort of "hostility-tag" game, making someone else "it." One Heart Wife who did makes a pretty good case for doing it. Incidentally, she illustrates how meaningless your husband's temporary hostility toward you really is:

> My brother-in-law was with me, endlessly. And I was most hostile toward him. I just took it all out on him, I guess.
>
> I'm very fond of him. But if you have one person to be hostile with, maybe that's good. Maybe you shouldn't feel guilty about it too much. It helps, it really does!
>
> I mean, there's just nothing you can do, so it helps to have someone to just blow off at!
>
> I guess everybody needs somebody to be hostile with.

Probably. We are certainly not urging you to play hostility-tag (and do not make the children "it," whatever you do!); but you should not feel too horrid if you find yourself flying off the handle during this period.

There is one more reason you can expect to be the target of

your husband's hostility. And this probably runs the deepest
and hurts the most.

He does feel guilty about what he has "done" to you and the
shambles he feels he's made of your life, the "dirty deal" he has
given you. So . . . he turns on the person "making" him feel
guilty. It is a hard thing to be the object of hostility that is born,
at least in part, of guilt feelings toward you. But isn't that quite
often the reason for hostility?

What can you do about his personality change and his hostility?

You have already done the most important thing: you have
found out that it is liable to happen. We asked the Heart Wife
who had asked herself "Why *me*" this question: "If you'd only
had someone to talk to, and if you knew about the hostility ahead
of time, would it have made it easier for you?" Her answer was,

> Ohhh . . . yes! As Dr. Spock says, *this* is typical of age eighteen
> months, *this* is typical of two years. If someone had said, *this* is
> typical of a heart attack, I could have taken . . . *anything!*
>
> Just like you can take it with the baby!

That is what you can do. Take it—and take it easy. Understand it. Realize it is temporary. Do not panic, do not retaliate.
Wait him out. As soon as he is up, off his back, figuratively and
literally, he will find other messages for his life than the one he
thinks he sees written on the ceiling.

CHAPTER
9

Heart Patience

There is only one thing we can tell you with even a pretense of firm, confident authority about how long coronary patients stay in the hospital: it varies. In fact, even *that* varies! Some doctors inflexibly keep their heart patients in the hospital a minimum length of time.

The amount of time heart patients stay in hospitals depends on so many variables, there is nothing even vaguely approaching a meaningful average. Especially since one factor is what theory your doctor likes best.

Theories change. Fifty years ago, doctors were positive the slightest strain on an infarcted heart was next door to suicide. So patients were routinely confined to bed, as nearly immobile as possible, for *six months*. Today, a cardiologist is more likely to ask himself not "How long must this patient stay in bed to be on the safe side?" but "How fast can we safely get him up and around, then back home?" There is no medical disagreement over the advantages of getting patients home quickly, only over what minimum time in the hospital is safe.

Of course, your interest in bed-rest theories of modern medicine is limited. All you really want to know is how long your husband will have to stay in the hospital. The point is not only that we cannot give you the slightest clue (which is no surprise) but that at the start of your husband's hospital stay (outside the CCU), even the doctor can give you only the sketchiest notion. A moment's reflection tells you why. Release from the CCU marks the definite end of heart damage from the attack, but only the beginning of healing. The doctor wants to be sure the healing is coming along satisfactorily before he will let your husband go far from the hospital's emergency-coping facilities. If he is willing to hazard so much as a rough guess, it will be in terms of "between such and such a number of weeks," with an ample enough spread to keep you from being unhappy and him from looking foolish if there are modifications in either direction.

So you may be sorely tempted to extrapolate from the experience of others an idea as to how long *your* husband will be in the hospital.

We would like to give you some advice in the matter. Don't.

DO NOT COMPARE NOTES WITH OTHER HEART WIVES AS TO YOUR HUSBAND'S PROGRESS OR FORECASTS AS TO LENGTH OF STAY IN THE HOSPITAL. DO NOT TRY TO FIGURE OUT HOW LONG IT WILL BE BY AVERAGING THE LENGTH OF TIME OTHER MEN STAY.

We give every Heart Wife that advice. To our best knowledge, it has never yet been followed. It is not humanly possible to find out that Mr. A went home in two weeks, Mr. B in seventeen days, Mr. C in three weeks—and not feel awful if your husband is still in the hospital on the twenty-second day. We can nod our heads and say we understand that each case is so different, and with so many imponderables (including various pet theories of individual cardiologists), that length of stay in the hospital is almost no guide to how severe one heart attack is compared to another, and absolutely unconnected to a prognosis of smoothness, ease, or completeness of recovery. Yes-yes-yes, but . . . And then it starts: "Your husband is going home tomorrow? But he came into the CCU two days after my husband. What isn't the doctor telling us!"

Conversely, it is impossible to feel entirely chipper about

your husband going home in three weeks when you know Mr. Z stayed four weeks, then had a relapse or another attack the day he went home. Doesn't that doctor know he's had a heart attack? Why, he's treating it like some splinter you remove and mommy-kiss and go on home and forget the whole thing!

You see? Either way you lose. So why play?

Because it is nearly impossible not to, that's why. Still, it is only *nearly* impossible; so we keep on advising Heart Wives not to trade progress reports. Maybe you will be the first to follow it. Or at least the first who absolutely refuses to let herself make the painful mistake of thinking "how long" equals "how severe."

You have other things to think about. There are so many things you should get done during the period of your husband's hospital recovery, however long it is will not be too much time.

You are cutting a pattern for a new life-style. And your basic material is the fabric of your relationship with your husband. Up to now you may have the impression from our discussion that it is one crisis after another, with him sulking or shouting, hostile or glum. That is a built-in danger with any discussion of problems, because problems are so vivid. You may come to feel your whole role, and the key to successfully surviving, is to cope with problems as they crop up. In truth, it is hard not to take this fireman's approach to what you do as a Heart Wife. When your husband is unaccountably hostile toward you, when he is denying his heart attack and defiantly searching out "safe" rules to break, your thinking tends to be along lines of, "Now how am I going to handle *this* mess!" You are trying so hard to avoid or minimize unpleasant incidents, there just does not seem to be time or energy left for thinking beyond the moment. That is true for every Heart Wife at this stage.

Even so, it is vital that you keep before you at least the image of your real goal. Not stopgap solutions to take-them-as-they-come problems, but a lasting (if ever-modifying) solution to the Big Problem of helping your husband (and yourself) establish a new life-style.

We do not like the term "life-style." We use it because we

cannot think of a less trendy phrase that describes what we are talking about as well. And it does suggest a total program or plan for living, one in which many different facets of your relations with your husband and your family come into play. Since this is a particularly momentous time in establishing that pattern, and since you truly cannot plot out each move you make to fit into the pattern, you must fall back on a general guideline for what to do in most situations and the way to do it.

Call it . . . attitude.

It is the key to knowing you are doing the right thing in your reaction to the many quirks and stresses of your husband's behavior while he is in the hospital. It is also the key to establishing a sensible foundation on which you and he will build your new life-style. It starts with a realization of what your husband needs and how his needs affect what he does and says.

A psychiatrist had this to say about the psychological needs of any man at this stage of coronary recovery:

Dr.: It's an ultimate question. He asks himself, "Is there anyone I can really depend on, or do I have to continue to be . . . Superman. The only way I'm not Superman is by being sick—really near death. That's the only time I'm adequately taken care of."

H.W.C.: But . . . isn't it wrong for us to encourage that feeling? Of being rewarded for being sick?

Dr.: But the wife *does* encourage it—by not *doing* the "taking care of." Just as a natural, routine thing—only a little more intense, right now.

But there has to be a way of presenting it so it is not demeaning to his self-respect and his self-esteem. Because to such men it is very important to be responsible and not to lean on others.

So the question is how can she work something out that can be mutually acceptable to both of them? It really requires a major reorientation—on both their parts.

His reorientation will have to come along in a while. But how long a while, how complete and useful it is, may depend in large measure on you and your reactions right now. Your attitude must be one of *constructive* understanding; you must realize the sort of blow the heart attack has been to his entire self-image, how enormous a blow it has been, and how much he needs to feel that your sole interest now is in his need. Automatically applying that test—"What does he need"—in determining your words and actions (and your reaction to his) during this critical period will show you how to make him know he is loved and needed, make him aware of how sensitive you are to his feelings, make him know you know how he feels about himself right now (and, by extension, how you disagree with his temporary self-downgrading). Finally, you will make him see that you feel he is entirely entitled to be taken care of for a while.

At any particular moment, you may be hard-pressed to see the relevance of the guideline to your actions. That is why we say the key must be your attitude—the basic stuff of which your words and actions are made. If you are headed in the right directions, you cannot go far wrong, even in the little things.

No one is smart enough, and no one has time enough, to ponder every little word and act. You simply have to let yourself be guided by a continually operating instinct. And it is that instinct we mean by "attitude."

See how it works. Here is how two different Heart Wives handled what amounts to an almost identical situation.

The first Heart Wife told us:

> He wanted clean pajamas everyday—*every* day. And if I didn't bring him clean pajamas, or if I skipped a day, or something like that, and he had to wear the same pajamas, he was very annoyed with me. "What the hell did I have to do with my time that I couldn't get him his clean pajamas?"

That seems like a fairly routine little transaction. Demanding, unreasonable husband, totally oblivious to his wife's feelings, trampling on her until she rebels. Then we have another case:

I got him two large pairs of boxer shorts—that he could slip on. And we played the game of "I took them home and washed them and brought a clean pair back, everyday." I could have gotten him six pair. But, nope, that would have upset him—so I didn't.

Now, that is another matter. Here we seem to have a clearly "rooster-pecked" little wife, meek and subservient even to demands on her time and energy that might be textbook examples of the unreasonable and unnecessary. Objectively now, doesn't it seem that way?

Well, things are not what they seem. There may have been plenty of substantial reasons for the first Heart Wife to be disgruntled about her relationship with her husband; but his asking for fresh pajamas everyday cannot be counted among them. The fact is, she actually did *not* have all that much to do with her time. She surely could have arranged it. In fact, we suspect she did not once "forget" them! More likely, she painstakingly remembered . . . *not* to bring them.

And the "meek, subservient" wife? She is anything but that. Her own description of herself is: "I'm not exactly what you could call a 'shrinking-violet type'—I've led an interesting life." Indeed she has! She is a professional woman whose day is full-to-bursting with activities, which neither stopped nor even diminished while her husband was in the hospital.

The difference between the two women and how they handled their similar situations comes down to attitude. The second Heart Wife realized that this was no time for a "rational" approach. Of course her husband did not "need" to save the cost of four pairs of shorts. But he did need her to play that "washing shorts" game; he needed signs that she cared and wanted to please him and take care of him.

Attitude influences what you do and what you don't do. For example, take another set of Heart Wives, again approaching the same sort of problem.

The first one of them had never learned to drive and now deeply regretted the fact; it meant that while her husband was in the hospital, she would either have to take taxis, which were expensive, or impose on friends and relatives for rides. But, most of all (she told us wistfully), how nice it would be if she could drive her husband places before he had the doctor's permission to do the driving, himself. What's more, she was worried about who would drive him somewhere in an emergency.

The other Heart Wife knew how to drive—and wished she didn't. She admitted that she was a poor driver; she avoids it whenever she can. And she contemplated the idea of chauffeuring her husband with an apprehension edging toward downright terror. Her driving had always made him nervous, and now she was afraid one of her typical screeching stops or near-misses might bring on another heart attack.

Objectively, the solution to both problems is the same: learn to drive. The first Heart Wife went to considerable trouble to arrange for lessons. Driving schools are fairly expensive, and the first couple was on a tight budget. So she got a friend of her husband's to teach her, making elaborate changes in her schedule to fit his.

The second Heart Wife was content to simply carry on at rather tedious length about how she "dreaded the day" when she would have to drive her poor husband. Touching concern, huh?

Knowing nothing more about these two sets of couples, whose chances do you like better for full, fast recovery with easy transition and adjustment to a new life-style?

We have no reason to think one wife loved her husband more than the other loved hers. The wives with what we consider the wrong attitude do not love their husbands any less than the other two wives love theirs. But they were unwilling or unable to translate whatever degree of love they felt (and it may very well have been considerable) into constructive action. We imagine it was because their attitudes did not let them perceive a need for action. The wrong attitude came from looking only at the objective situation: the one husband did not "need" fresh pajamas each and every day, come what may; the other husband could have easily afforded a professional chauffeur. Neither saw how much their husbands *did* need some things to be indulged. Unreasonably maybe; but isn't that what "indulging" someone means? The other wives certainly thought so. Their attitude was "What will make my husband happy and comfortable?" It was not boxer shorts or driving lessons; it was a wife who would take pains to please him.

In this area, attitude need have nothing at all to do with reality. The solutions you come up with, in every case, if motivated by the right attitude, cannot help but be "right." Even if, on their face, they are not realistic solutions to practical problems at all. They solve something much more important: the problem of how your husband feels about himself, about you, about how you evidently feel about him and about the future of your relationship.

When we nag about the need to consult your husband, we are really talking about attitude. It is the attitude that you care about his wishes—and, more, letting him know you do—that is important. In fact, you will find the right attitude much more helpful than any suggestion we can make as to things you should get done before your husband comes home. With the proper attitude you will be proceeding along the right path. The rest is detail.

Still, you do have to take care of details. So we'll take a look at them in the following chapter.

CHAPTER

10

More Decisions
(A Slightly More Expanded
Checklist)

Like the last checklist, this will remind you of things to take care of. However, now we are in an area where a good many of the problems and the decisions you should make involve situations that you will face later on in the course of your husband's recovery. That means that a somewhat fuller discussion is necessary so you can see clearly what is involved and can head off problems before they occur.

Stay loose—and start checking:

Education / Information

There is so much to learn about so many things, it is easy to become appalled and decide that, since you cannot learn it all anyway, you might as well just drift along, picking up what you absolutely must know along the way. That is not a good idea. "On-the-job" training is a distinctly hard way to be a Heart Wife. We could try to be inspirational and repeat the old proverb about a journey of a thousand miles beginning with a single step. But that never did seem too comforting a thought; after that single step, you are still a depressingly long way from the end. Especially since, in this case, there is no end to what you will learn. Strangely enough, *that* is a comfort. The only reason for feeling intimidated by the volume of things you have to learn about is if you look at it as some fixed body of knowledge that must be mastered before it is useful—like a school subject to be learned for a final exam. It is not like that at all. It is more like learning to play a musical instrument, or speak a language or become a French chef. There is an inexhaustible store of things to learn, and learning them is a life's occupation. But just because you may never know everything about the subject does not mean you cannot perform capably, even with passable eloquence, in relatively short order.

The reason to start learning now what you have to know later is not that you must start now or never learn what you should by the time your husband comes home. It is because the sooner you begin, the more fluent you will be in your practice of the various skills and more confident in your use of your knowledge as you go along, learning more all the while.

Here are the major areas you should know more about:

MEDICAL

Heart Wives who get most uptight about the doctors' orders, and who may have their whole families halfway up the wall with tension over those orders, are generally those who know the least about heart attacks and about what does and does not affect recovery from them. It is exactly like cooking. If you are like us, the first time you baked a cake all on your own, it was with recipe in hand and panic in heart lest a speck more or less of any ingredient, a degree of heat, a second of baking time ruin everything. Following rules is hard; applying rules you understand is much easier, in cooking, sewing, driving, any kind of job. And in being a Heart Wife, too.

To feel easy and comfortable in helping your husband follow the doctor's rules, you have to understand how the rules apply to a heart. That means you have to understand what makes a heart tick. The information we gave you in Chapter 2 is just a start toward understanding. We can recommend two books that helped us understand enough about the workings of the heart so that we could pass on to you a little information. Both books are so lucid we had no trouble following them (which is pretty high testimony to lucidity, our grasp of science being what it is). The books are *Heart Attack: New Hope, New Knowledge, New Life*, by Myron Prinzmetal, M.D. (Essandess, 1968), and *Heart Attack: You Don't Have to Die*, by Christaan Barnard, M.D. (Delacorte, 1972).

Unfortunately, we know of no book (including this one) that can do a total job of preparing you for what to expect in the way of unsettling physical reactions in the early stages of your husband's recovery. There are simply too many variables. You will feel less tense about everything, though, with every bit of increasing knowledge, including the knowledge that other Heart Wives have had the same unsettling experiences.

The most common one is, as one Heart Wife said,

> The first week he is home you wake up at all hours—five, six times, every night. And, you know, just look at him. Like, is he still . . . breathing?

It happens to nearly every Heart Wife. One woman compared it to the way a new mother "looks in on her baby five times a night—just checking." That is certainly true; but what is frightening is the fact that when you wake up, you may very well not be able to hear him breathe, and in panic decide he actually is not breathing. It has nothing to do with the heart attack; in a deep sleep, anyone's breathing becomes extremely shallow, often inaudible. You simply had no reason to notice before. Now you do. Perhaps *not* hearing anything was what woke you in the first place!

What can you do when it happens to you? Well, one Heart

Wife told us she put a mirror under her husband's nose to check up. You need not go that far. You can simply nudge him and see if he moves. Trouble is, that means taking a chance on waking him, which is not on the highly recommended list of cardiologists—or marriage counselors! Alternately, you can take our word for it that, yes, he is still breathing. If your husband were having another heart attack, you would know about it, even if he made no sound or movement, the same way you "knew" he "wasn't breathing." Call it mental telepathy, or just call it being married. You would know.

We said *nearly* every Heart Wife has the experience. Ironically, those who have exactly the opposite experience are even more frightened:

> Nobody told me there was still fluid and that when he was sleeping at night he was going to sound "rattley." Nobody told me that! So I was awake three nights, listening to each breath, inhale and exhale.

How come nobody told her? Because nobody knew it was going to happen. The condition she described is known as "rales." It does not develop very often; it is an indication that the heart is not compensating enough, leaving a little blood in the lungs with each beat. It should be taken care of—and can be, easily—but it is not very serious, disappearing of its own accord with rest.

Why don't doctors automatically give Heart Wives a rundown on things that may happen? Three reasons. First, there would never be time enough for a doctor to go into all the possible variations of physiological reactions; second, the doctor has no way of knowing which reactions any particular Heart Wife will find frightening; third, the doctor may not even know about a wife's psychological reaction to certain physical facts about a heart patient, unless the doctor is a woman whose husband has had a heart attack, that is.

Of course, even if you knew everything about a heart attack, you would still worry about your husband. But it is certain that the more you know about what is normal in the course of coronary recovery, the better prepared you will be to take things in stride.

The best source of information is your husband's doctor. Unhappily, he is also the least accessible source. Most Heart Wives we talk to complain sooner or later about not being able to get in touch with the doctor nearly often enough to ask all the questions on their minds. There are two solutions to that problem. The first is, make the most of the time you do get with him, be prepared with questions you want to ask. That means writing them down as they occur to you and having the list with you when you see the doctor or call him.

A Heart Wife describes the second solution:

> Well, I write the doctor letters. I tell him, "I know you can't answer the telephone always, and I want 'X' question answered."
>
> When we go in, he always tells my husband, "Your wife wrote me a letter." This pleases my husband—that I take the trouble. And it gets us answers!

Better, clearer, more considered answers, we expect! A letter gives the doctor a chance to mull over your questions, instead of having to come up with Instant Genius while patients pile up in his waiting room.

If you have questions you feel cannot wait, be prepared to ask them in few enough words to leave with a nurse or answering service if the doctor is not immediately available. In general, you should find that the doctor will be more inclined to spend time when you want it if you are solicitous of his time when you can be.

Diet

You need two kinds of diet information: your doctor's specific diet restrictions or prescriptions for your husband and general information about shopping and cooking for heart patients. The first comes *only* from your doctor, and it totally overrules anything we—or anyone else—tell you. As for general information, the best sources are the American Heart Association and the American Dietary Association. In fact, the Heart Association has recently put together a total guide to coronary diet; it is called (reasonably enough) *The American Heart Association Cookbook* (David McKay, 1973). It is a must.

Four Heart Association pamphlets we have found particularly useful are "Recipes for Fat-controlled, Low-cholesterol Meals," "The Way to a Man's Heart (A Fat-controlled, Low-cholesterol Meal Plan to Reduce the Risk of Heart Attack)," "Available Products for the Controlled-fat Diet" and "Available Products for the Low-Sodium Diet." All four should be available at the nearest chapter of the American Heart Association, without charge. (If no office is listed in your phone book, write the head office, at 44 East 23rd Street, New York, New York 10010.) The first does not have many recipes. Nevertheless, this pamphlet is valuable for its viewpoint; it helps you get the hang of the principles of low-calorie and low-fat cooking, which we will explore in depth in Chapter 19. The second pamphlet gives you, in very handy chart form, the foods that are and are not approved for heart patients *in general.* The third and fourth are really shopping guides, listing foods by brand names that are generally all right and those that are dangerous for heart patients.

The American Dietary Association has available at nominal charge (50¢ apiece, mostly, but with a $2 minimum order) reprints from the *ADA Journal.* They are ponderous reading, but you do pick up an amazingly large amount of information from them. The Publications Department, 620 North Michigan Avenue, Chicago, Illinois 60611, will send you a list of those available.

To show how important it is to check with your doctor for any special dietary factors in your husband's case (as opposed, that is, to heart patients in general), both organizations offer meal-planning guides for fat- and sodium-restricted diets. However . . . *a doctor's prescription is required for them.* They do not include medicine, but no one should just concoct a diet, however sound it may be according to general rules, without particular reference to a particular patient's needs. And only your doctor is qualified to determine those.

Things to Find Out

In addition to what you should start learning, there are various facts—and figures—you should start to find out about now in order to make a number of decisions that are better made sooner than later. The sooner you start, the less turmoil later on.

For instance, do you know where your family stands financially? What do you have in the way of savings? Investments? Property? Will your husband's income continue while he is in the hospital? While resting at home? If so, for how long? If not, do you have other sources of income? And is there anything that must be done now to make sure the income actually comes in? Are there insurance claims to file? State Disability or Workmen's Compensation?

Do you have a specific budget? If your income will be different from what it was before the heart attack, your budget may have to change to make the money last until your husband is back at work. If you do not already operate on a set family budget, can you figure one out, or should you ask for help? (This is something you probably should *not* consult your husband about; at least not until you are sure he is only minimally despondent about his future.)

If finances are obviously going to be a tight problem, should you get a job? Or if you already have one, should you be looking for one that pays more?

These questions may be worrisome now; but better worry now than panic when the money runs out!

If you need help with any of the questions, the hospital social-services people can either help or direct you to the relevant state or county office.

If your husband's occupation makes it unlikely that he will be able to return to it (heavy physical labor, high-risk work, etc.), now is the time to begin planning. What kind of work can he do when he is ready to go back to work? Talk it over with him. You have a powerful weapon on your side that, used correctly, can result in your husband ending up in a *better* job because of the attack. It is probably true that employers are generally leery of promoting men who have had heart attacks. At the same time, those employers just as likely feel some guilt. "We let him overwork; he drove himself too hard—for *us!*" Beyond that, there is the question of company morale. Fire a man when he has had a heart attack? Monstrous! And companies, like people, do not generally care to be thought monsters. So even if, in fact, they are monsters, they will keep him on—at least "until he gets back on his feet," as the formula goes. However, if your husband has taken the trouble to think where he could actually do a useful job (after a realistic inventory of his abilities and the company's needs), and has set out to qualify himself for that job, the company's management almost has to let him try. As we said in the previous chapter, this is a nation that admires winners; but we are absolutely *wild* about anyone who shows he intends to come back and win after being flat on his back. Now, your husband is not "flat on his back" (except literally—which does not mean a thing in this case); but they do not know that. They will give him full credit. So start finding out how to cash in on it as soon as possible.

Again, the social-services office at the hospital should be able to assist, if only in steering you toward the kind of help you need: a state or county rehabilitation or retraining program, a high school extension program, etc.

If your husband is near the age at which retirement is a plausible life-style, this might be a fine time to discuss it. To aid in your thinking, you might consult the nearest office of the Social Security Administration about what benefits you can expect (assuming your husband does not already have a pension in store). Remember, though, that retirement is often a tricky subject under any circumstances; many men regard it with apprehension. So give it considerable thought before suggesting it. In fact, you probably should not mention it unless you had discussed retirement plans with enthusiasm before the heart attack.

Keeping Him Happy

The greatest enemy to your husband's morale in the hospital is time. There is so much of it! And you must play a constantly increasing role in filling the time: you start to be responsible for other people's visits (which also means other people's *non*visits when you have reason to feel some are too frequent, too long, too upsetting, or otherwise too taxing on your husband).

To complicate matters, how things go now can affect how they go later.

As an example, there is the problem of the children.

Your husband misses them; they miss him. The young adults are not much problem; they can come visit. But many hospitals will not allow infants or youngsters to visit. Hospitals can be dangerous for children, whose resistance to disease is usually lower than that of adults, while some adults, especially when sick, have a pretty low resistance to noise and tumult, both of which children have been known to cause for minimum reason and with no warning. If your husband's hospital bars children, you must do something to mitigate the pain of separation—especially since it is under circumstances so frightening to both sides.

Consider the objective facts from the youngsters' point of view. Their father has disappeared; he must be desperately sick, or why would he be away so long? There is nothing they can do about it; and they are singled out as the only ones not allowed to see him (unlike, say, their older brothers and sisters, their aunts and uncles, seemingly everyone in the world!).

Are we getting a touch hysterical over the situation? If you explain things to them, won't that be all right?

Probably not. It helps, but after you have explained why they cannot go see their father to four- or five- or even ten-year olds, how will that change the appearance of the facts we have outlined? Precious little.

If possible, your husband's reaction is even more complex. Whatever guilt he feels about you has an exact counterpart in the guilt he feels about what he has done to his children. He is worried about making them *feel* deserted, useless, scared, set apart and all the rest. This is on top of the fairly hallucinatory worries we discussed in the last chapter about how he can clothe and educate them—or even enjoy them—once he is out of the hospital.

This is one problem, though, you can solve with stunning economy, since what makes him happy will go a long way toward making them happy, too.

Here are the most effective measures we have run across.

One Heart Wife had her children write poems and letters and draw pictures for their father everyday. Everyone's favorite was the portrait: themselves helping mother, mother getting ready to go to the hospital, father getting a good rest in bed so he can come home as soon as possible.

At the other end, she picked up little souvenirs to bring home every few days: real, live plastic *hospital* straws; postcards showing the hospital with an X marking The Room. (Pick any window. Accuracy is for surveyors and cat burglars.) Every now and then she took them a pack of Life Savers or chewing gum—direct from father, with a note. For a special treat, about once a week, there was a special surprise from the hospital gift shop. *What* they send him or he sends them does not much matter: anything will serve as a constant reminder that one thinks of, misses, and loves the other. It is the hospital straw's finest hour!

A little more elaborate (and a little more expensive) reminders are pictures and recordings. A Polaroid camera has the most immediacy; but it does cost more, and so does film for it. But any pictures with any camera are wonderful!

So are tape recordings. Cassette tape recorders are the

simplest, and can be bought for as little as $20. Tape for them is a minor expense and can be used over and over again.

VISITORS

For quite a while we thought the only important points about visitors were negative: not letting them all come at once—"feast or famine," as one patient put it—getting rid of those who stay too long, banning any whose visits upset your husband.

Then, in the course of a post-hospital meeting, one ex-patient told us:

> There's another side to that, you know. If no one comes in to see you, you start to wonder who's keeping them out? And why? Am I worse than they're telling me? So bad, I can't have any visitors?

It is surely a point to keep in mind. And one way you can help is by making sure friends and relatives do visit in a regular, spaced-out schedule.

However, if your husband has too many visitors, if he is not getting the rest he should, ask the doctor to specify the correct number of visitors, week-by-week. Then schedule visits accordingly.

You will still have problems. The first may seem to be one of selection. Most Heart Wives begin by being afraid there are going to be hurt feelings among his friends. If the doctor says one visitor, and your husband decides on Charlie, won't Joe be hurt? And how about Aunt Mabel? Actually, this turns out to be more a theoretical than a practical problem.

One Heart Wife told us that because of complications, her husband had been in the CCU nearly a month. When he was sent to a regular room, the doctors felt he needed rest more than he needed company. As a result, this Heart Wife ended up with nearly all the possible combinations of visitor problems:

> When they cut him off altogether, I said, "You're making a mistake." I sat down with the cardiologist and our regular doc-

tor, and I said, "My husband needs people. Not scads of people, but he does need some of his friends. It's very important."

Finally they said, "Okay, but only a few." Well, I simply said "no" to most and "yes" to the few he really wanted. When your husband's health is at stake, it's easy!

Besides, I could put the whole thing off on the doctors. I told the people I had to turn down that the doctors had said *no* visitors—and I didn't volunteer information. I didn't run around saying "Rocky got to see him." And I told Rocky, "Don't go telling everybody you saw him."

And you find out that the true friends would completely understand. I felt a little guilty when someone called and said, "So-and-so said that so-and-so got to see him—and how come?" I merely said, "So-and-so was allowed in because so-and-so happens to be his closest friend."

I don't think I was rude; but I didn't have time to indulge my friends' trivialities. I just didn't have time for it.

Every Heart Wife we know would endorse that outlook and those actions. Especially her point about those friends who do *not* seem willing or able to understand. No one has time for those "trivialities."

As for the friends who were nice and did understand and did not insist that they be allowed to see her husband, the Heart Wife told them:

"In a couple of weeks you'll all be able to see him." Meanwhile, I had all of his friends writing him letters. Because it was very important that he still feel there was contact with the outside world. And you have no idea how happy his friends were to write the letters—and how thrilled he was, everyday, to be reading scads of letters!

He would write little notes back, and his friends were as delighted as he was!

After a while, visiting is likely to approach open-house proportions. That is when scheduling to avoid the "feast or famine" pattern gets to be important, but not essential, due to the built-in limits of hospital room size and hospital rules that generally limit the number of visitors at one time. Plus the disinclination of doctors to conduct business in a convention atmosphere. The simplest way to handle scheduling is with an appointment calendar. Except you should not be the one who handles it. Nor should your husband. (We will discuss who should, and why, in the next section of this chapter.) But you definitely should discuss the idea of the calendar with your husband, letting him decide on frequency among those friends and relatives who have said they would like to visit as often as possible or can be expected to want to. There are two important reasons your husband should not do the actual scheduling: The first is that he should not feel that he has to "keep a book" on people's friendship, or that, by saying no, he is the one disappointing people who are, after all, giving an expression of their concern and friendship by wanting to visit. The second reason is to preserve for him the element of pleasant surprise when each visitor walks in the door.

ACTIVITIES

Of course, "keeping him happy" means more than visitors. It means a certain amount of activity. There will be two kinds: either "entertainment" (perhaps distraction would be a better word) or morale-building.

The most usual sorts of entertainment are TV and light reading, whatever sort he has always liked. But you might try to provide some supplementary entertaining activity.

What sort depends on what interests him, and what you think might. Our suggestions are only a starter set for your own imagination. Would he get absorbed in puzzles? Jigsaw, crossword, chess, bridge, that sort? Is there something he has always had a hankering to do in the way of reading and never had the distraction-free time for? Like reading all of *War and Peace* or the collected works of Shakespeare or Dickens? Naturally, any portable hobbies he has are a godsend. And if he ever thought he might be interested in some, now is the time to try.

Morale-building activities may seem the same as the entertainment types at first glance. That is the rather sneaky beauty of them: you may be able to get him interested in them without him feeling that you are pushing. Each stresses the future.

For instance, we mentioned puzzles. Crossword puzzles can beguile an hour or so; the same goes for bridge or chess problems. The difference is that anyone can do a crossword puzzle, but only those who already know how to play bridge or chess can do problems. This might be a wonderful time for your husband to learn bridge or chess, or any other game that requires skill and technique: pinochle, gin rummy, backgammon, whatever. It is also a great chance to improve his skill. If he has a regular poker or pinochle game with the boys, get him a couple of books by experts on the game's theory. He can steal a march, "flat on his back," and come back a better player.

The point is, he is learning something of use *for the future,* thinking in terms of a future in which he can do something he was not able to do before.

How much better morale builder can there be!

Depending on what sort of person your husband is, he might prefer more heavyweight self-improvement. If there is something he always thought might be useful for him to know, accounting, business law, stock-investment strategy—anything that can be learned from books, in fact—this is a perfect time for him to start learning. And even more than with the entertainment skills, this is a token of belief in a future that can be even better than the past.

Of course, there is also his present, immediate morale to consider. One Heart Wife hit on the happy idea of bringing all household expense checks for her husband to make out and sign. They had a joint account, and she had normally paid the bills; this was her way of showing him he was still a thoroughgoing part of his family's existence, heart attack or no.

Nurses

No matter how much time you plan to be at the hospital, your husband will not see as much of you as he does of the nurses. You will not have the opportunity to take care of him as much as they will, just in terms of sheer hours of the day when nurses are there and you are not.

And the chances are overwhelming that they will take very good care of your husband indeed. The fact is, every woman who has volunteered information on the subject has said things like, "The nurses spoiled him rotten," and "They really went all-out for him" or some such; each was convinced that her husband was so cute and so lovable and so brave, the nurses gave him the kind of treatment reserved for heads of state, the immediate family of that hospital's Chief of Medicine, and the dreamier movie stars.

Nonetheless, everyone involved—you, your husband, the nurses—are human beings. And it is only human to do that little extra for people you like. In theory, of course, a nurse is a professional who will unstintingly give her all, irrespective of personal feelings. In practice, whom do you want taking care of your husband, a friend—or someone whose personal involvement ranges between indifference and dislike?

And even if someone were to show us absolute proof that it didn't matter, we would still want to go out of our way to make friends of the nurses, to engage their sympathy and interest on behalf of our husbands.

There are any number of ways to do it, the best being whatever comes most naturally to you. After all, you will only be expressing a genuine feeling of friendliness and appreciation for people who are seeing that your husband is comfortable and is getting the care and rest he needs. Here is what one Heart Wife did:

I introduced myself to the nurses, and I told them all, "This is a very dear, sweet, special human being—and we're madly in love with each other, and I want you to give him extra special care." And I went into the gift shop, and I brought back a bunch of cookies and candy, and I said, "Just to remind you how sweet *he* is!"

Her attitude, demonstrated and expressed, was one that made the nurses care about the couple and about the patient.

There is another, tougher point about her tangible evidence of appreciation to the nurses. Giving money is generally considered inappropriate (unless you have a private nurse, of course), or professionally infra dig. But gifts are fine. If they are homey things, a cake, cookies, fudge you have made, all the better, but stuff from the gift shop is fine, too. Don't think of it as a bribe or tip or anything like that; it will make things awkward. Just treat it as an expression of thoughtful gratitude.

Understand, it is not at all necessary. They are taking care of your husband, not holding him for ransom. But if it feels right, do it! If you bake brownies and take some to the nurses, they will be touched by the thought—even if they are on diets!

Another excellent way to make the nurses care about you is to show an interest in them. A Heart Wife was explaining to us that she got the most lonely and miserable and worried at night. So she would call the hospital. (Incidently, it is perfectly all right to call at any hour. Ask for the charge nurse on your husband's floor and simply ask how he is. They will not wake him to find out; but it is comforting to hear someone right there on the floor say he is fine.)

> I decided he's going to be here a long time, so I might as well establish a good relationship with the nurses so they wouldn't say, you know, "Oh, God! not her again!"
>
> This is important, because I've seen some wives who become real nuisances to the nurses.
>
> I'd call sometimes when I'd wake up, in the middle of the night. And I'd talk to the nurse, and say, "How are you, Connie?" and, "Gee! Your hair looked nice today, and is everything with the husband okay?" I felt as though I had a relationship going with her, too, which made it easier for me.

That kind of relationship *will* make "it" (calling late at night; asking nurses to do something; practically *anything)* easier. And you will feel all the more assured that your husband is being taken care of by people who do care. Personally.

Your Social Life

Can your husband say the same about you?

He should be able to. He should know that you are being taken care of, too. At least a little bit. Because the more lonely and unhappy he thinks you are, the worse he will feel, and the guiltier. In the normal course of things, you are going to be miserably unhappy—and show it! Here are notes we took at one of the first in-hospital Heart Wife meetings we conducted when we were just getting the program under way.

> Mrs. _____ said that she sleeps with a transistor radio going all night. Finds this somewhat comforting. Eats just anything (sometimes nothing) for dinner. Can't concentrate—just listens to the radio . . . not interested in TV, crossword puzzles, or knitting, all of which interested her while her husband was at home. Friends and relatives have all invited her for dinner, but she doesn't feel like going, feels she is not good company, therefore nobody would like to be around her.

And from the same meeting:

> Major concern of Mrs. _____ is lack of consideration and apparent insincerity of most of her friends. All said "Isn't there *something* I can do for you while your husband is in the hospital," several offered to drive her back and forth *sometime*. Offer was made, then that was the last she heard from most of them. Felt hurt and disappointed, that as long as she gave "lavish dinner parties and invited them to fancy places," she had many friends, but now look! Said she'd have been happy if one of them would just drop by, without all the fuss of asking "when?" Like Mrs. _____ [above], expressed how lonely it is to go home to an empty apartment . . . eating irregularly, too; sleeping poorly; also finds it hard to concentrate.

That was a major theme at nearly all meetings, and with a majority of Heart Wives. You probably feel down in the dumps, too.

Sure, it would be nice if you were at your scintillating best right now (nice but strange). It would be grand if you could stay cheerful through it all. Some Heart Wives do manage through conscious, painstaking effort:

> My friends were very helpful—and I tried to be brave and, you know, cute and funny and helpful so they wouldn't worry that I was collapsing or anything.

Some can; most can't. And even those who can, you notice, need a lot of help from their friends.

Don't be hard on them. People do not generally offer unless they mean it. Make up a list—mentally, or on paper—of things various friends reasonably could do for you if they ask. And when they ask, tell them. All but the closest friends will have a fear of intruding on your worry and will hesitate to jump into things without your specific permission. And remember that when they invite you somewhere, it is not because they expect you to provide merriment to a dinner; it is because of their concern for a friend's well-being.

As for being rotten company—well, if you feel anything like we felt, you probably are; so wouldn't it be kind of pleasant to be around people who are good company for a while? You will be doing them a favor by letting them feel they are helping. And by taking you out of yourself for a while, they will be helping your husband, too.

One Heart Wife summed up the situation exactly:

> My friends would come to the hospital and take me for lunch. And my husband was pleased at the fact that I had not cut my life off.

Among the friends who will ask what they can do, some will be closer than others. If, among the particularly close ones, a couple of them stand out as good organizers, people who enjoy taking care of things, the answer to them should be "Yes! you can save my life—or my sanity, at any rate."

What they can do is act as clearing house for visitors and for chauffeur-dinner-companions. We know how much it can mean, because it was done for us. Friends took over the scheduling. They kept a calendar; whenever anyone called about visiting, we would refer them to our friends. There was no problem at all about transportation: if a would-be visitor did not or could not drive, our friends let us know and that day we did the picking up. Most of the time though, visitors came by for us. If we were going to be at the hospital most of the day, the "first shift" visitors (for the afternoon visiting hours) would pick us up, and the evening visitors would take us home.

That is pretty nearly an ideal situation.

If you cannot arrange for some friend to do it, do it yourself.

Work out a schedule so friends will drive you to the hospital on a given night and stop in for a visit. Invite the driving-friends to dinner (whether they take you, you take them, or it is Dutch Treat does not matter a bit). Don't be *bashful!* The people who ask you what they can do mean it (wouldn't you, in their place?). It is a kindness to them to give them something to do that will actually be of great value (be sure to let them know it!) to you and your husband. Be sure to let your husband know, too. He will appreciate the fact that friends are rallying around. It is flattering to him that they care and want to see he rests easy about you.

Putting Your House in Order

We do not mean that in an ominous way at all. Quite the opposite. Before your husband comes home, make a survey of your home to eliminate any potential hazards. Just as important, make any changes that will add to his comfort and the ease with which you take care of him. This is particularly important at first, when he will be largely confined to bed.

We suspect there is no such thing as an "ideal" layout. But we can show you how other Heart Wives have approached the problem; you can adapt the idea to your own setup.

One thing, though: make your arrangements (or re-arrangements) before your husband gets home; he should not feel that his homecoming is creating turmoil. And do not ask him whether he would like things rearranged for his greater comfort, just do it. Otherwise, you place him in the position of having to say, "Why sure, tear things apart for my comfort."

Actually, any arrangements you make may, more properly, come under the heading of adjustments. The way to arrive at them is simply to think about what your husband will probably be doing and where he will be doing it. That is what this Heart Wife did:

> I had a phone put in the living room because I knew he'd be in the living room more than he'd be in bed. He'd want to get back on his project, which would have been mostly on the phone anyhow. And he never did like business calls in bed. So I had it all set up as if it was his office—a corner of the living room—when he got home.

Simple. But effective. She knew her husband, knew what physical changes could be made that would make things easier for him—then made them.

Another Heart Wife made her survey and concluded there were some excellent reasons for simply turning one room into another:

> When you come into our house, there's this large family room with the kitchen on one side and the patio on the other. So I had them put the rented bed—an electric bed, so it was easier to sit up—I put it in the family room.
>
> It is a brighter, cheerier room than our bedroom. And if he wanted to sleep, he could always close the door and pull the drapes. Plus the fact that our house is "L" shape, and our bedroom is way at the other end.
>
> If I were in the kitchen, for example, I couldn't be talking constantly to him on the intercom; I would want him there, so he could have company.

During the day, when I was at work and the kids were at school, it was quiet. Which was fine. And the television was in that room, too.

When I came home, he could watch me in the kitchen, and the kids would want to sit down and talk with him—then they would go off and slide the door closed and they wouldn't disturb him.

It worked out fine!

Of course it did! She made it work out fine. As you will by looking around your home with an eye to arrangements that make sense—not to an architect, maybe, or to the editors of *House Beautiful,* but to you and your husband, and the rest of the family.

While we are on the subject of beds, the "rented bed" referred to was the hospital type; it is most handy for anyone who is going to be in bed for much of the day, during the better part of several weeks. The up-and-down back makes it fine for sitting up to read, watch TV, eat, visit—and even for getting in and out (though that really applies only for the extremely short period of time during which a patient is still worn out by the trip home and is still weak). You can rent one for about $160 a month. That is steep; but it is awfully convenient, if only for the first month home.

That brings up another thing you should *not* discuss with your husband. If whatever arrangements you think should be made will involve much in the way of expense, remember that every man who has a heart attack is afraid he will not be able to support his family the way he wants to, let alone pay for such luxuries as a little more comfort while he is in bed. If you decide he needs something, get it without asking him about it: he will either forbid squandering the money or he will worry about it.

That works both ways, of course. Since you realize how he feels about his earning power from now on, you must be able to say, in your own mind, that "yes"—whatever it is, you feel it is important enough to override what you know he would object to.

A personal instance: JoAnn and Forrest were both very

happy with, comfortable in, and proud of their home. The only problem was an almost Alpine-like flight of stairs up to the front door, a distinct disadvantage for the home of a heart patient fresh from the hospital. JoAnn was faced with the choice of moving (which she knew Forrest would hate) or spending a considerable amount of money to have a sort of monorail funicular put in. She was appalled by either choice. But, unlike you, she did not have the advantage of having someone to tell her what the effect would be—so she made the wrong decision. She discussed it with her husband. Wonderful! Now two people could agonize over the problem. The turning point came when Forrest came home. He had to be carried up the stairs. Predictably, he was deeply humiliated; here he was, a grown man, being carried up his own front steps. Today (when he walks up, jaunty as you please, and—infuriatingly—is not even breathing hard at the top) it would not bother him a bit. Then, it was a totally different matter. One look at his face and JoAnn decided no money in the bank was worth seeing him feeling what he was feeling.

It will not be for you, either.

There is a lot to decide, a lot to do. But with an attitude of caring and wanting to start your husband's ultimate recovery on the right track, the adjustment both of you will be making to each other and to your life, together, will be as easy and comfortable as possible. You will be able to do everything that is necessary and do it well—simply because that is what must be done. You may not always do things perfectly. Well, the patience we meant in the title of the last chapter refers to your attitude toward your husband. But it also applies to your attitude toward yourself. If you do the very best you can, you will be doing all that anyone can do. Be patient with your husband; be patient with yourself. And keep trying.

THE HOME

CHAPTER

11

A Home Is Not a Hospital

Nobody gets well in a hospital. Hospitals are conceived, designed, staffed, equipped and run to help people get better, not well. Once a patient is so much better that the only questions are how quickly and how thoroughly well he will get, he is packed off for home.

However, when the doctor says your husband is "ready to come home," he means *medically* ready. But is your husband psychologically ready? Is your home ready? Are you ready?

One woman we know was the enviable picture of Heart Wife cool throughout her husband's stay in the hospital. As she talked with us about the problems that had popped up, we were struck by the admirable calm and considered efficiency with which she dispatched each one. She simply did not make a wrong move. Then came the time when her husband was . . . ready.

> Suddenly it struck me, "I'm responsible!" I'm supposed to be doctor and nurses and dietician and all those modern machines, all in one. That's when I felt I really wasn't prepared. I panicked.

If *she* panicked, just imagine how her husband felt!

Now imagine how your husband feels.

There he is, about to be wrenched from the knowing care of professionals and delivered into the hands of amateurs. Worse still, the "chief of medicine" at the nonhospital to which he's going is fretful over her unreadiness to be of significant help in case he should need it.

It's a replay of the weaning anxiety he felt when about to leave the CCU. But with a number of important differences, both bad and good.

Let's start with the bad ones.

There was not much substance to his apprehension on leaving the CCU. Right down the corridor or clear across the hospital, he was still very close to help. And he was going to be monitored with particular diligence, whether in a formal coronary observation unit or not. The nurses knew all about the needs and dangers of the situation.

Now, no matter how close you live to a hospital, he is a phone call and an ambulance ride away from professional help. What's more, the speediest, most alert ambulance crew in the world will not come until called. Someone will have to phone. Suppose he is unconscious? Someone will have to notice his condition. But suppose "someone" is in the kitchen making dinner or on the phone or out shopping? And even after the call, what then? Suppose he needs help quickly, maybe before the ambulance gets there. Suppose the ambulance is delayed? Suppose . . .

But you get the idea. So let's move on to the good differences.

In the first place, your husband truly *is* ready to come home. And he feels it. He has not been this rested his entire adult life. He has eaten well—from a dietician's viewpoint, not a maître d's—and if necessary has lost weight. Aside from occasional contraband smuggled in by alleged "friends," he has given up anything remotely resembling bad health habits—smoking, drinking, overwork, and the like. And with you on the job, he has had an absolute minimum of extraneous worries. He feels great. Positively terrific! And . . . oh, yes, bored silly. As one husband said,

No question—I was ready! How I knew was, for the last ten days, all I could think about was sex.

Boy! was I well!

Boy! was he wrong! People do not get well in hospitals. But a coronary patient characteristically has an illusion of extreme physical well-being at this point. He will find out how weak he is shortly, when just the effort of coming home leaves him drained. But right now feeling fine helps allay his apprehension. When he moved from the CCU, the pain and terror of the attack were only days past; now he has been feeling splendid for weeks. It helps.

So does the near banality of his surroundings. His apprehension upon leaving the CCU had nothing to do with the actual room; he was anxious about leaving the equipment and personnel. He was physically attached and dependent on the dazzling array of CCU equipment one minute, the next minute they were nowhere in sight. Neither were the CCU specialists. By now, it has been weeks since he has seen monitors, IVs, defibrillators, or anything more elaborate than the already familiar blood-pressure sphygmomanometer and the overly familiar (anyway you look at it) rectal thermometer. And the nurses, lately, have not been called upon to display any greater technical virtuosity than you would expect in a good waitress, much less a good wife!

So, to balance the fact that the help he associates with a hospital is farther away, the specifics that make it a hospital—as opposed to merely an outrageously overpriced and far from first-class hotel—those things are equally far away in time and his immediate experience.

Yet, for all of that, he will be apprehensive. He will be anxious about what kind of help he may get, if he needs it. He will be nervous about how competent the care at home is likely to be. He may not feel that way in this moment of anticipation. But when he is home and discovers how weak he is, what a long road it is to being truly well—that is when the anxieties start. "Suppose . . ." And you can do nothing about it.

If that sounds defeatist, we mean it to. We want to forestall the two most common mistakes Heart Wives make at this point.

The first is to turn your home into a hospital, complete with a nurse. He needs the normal, easy relaxation—and, yes, even normal stresses—of home. For a heart patient, getting well means adjusting to a normal life in a normal home. The more "successfully" you turn your home into a hospital and yourself into a hospital attendant, the worse it is for your husband's recovery.

He needs you, his wife, not a nurse, doctor or heart monitor. You need him, your husband, not a patient. You will both resent a continuation of his role as a patient for one second longer than necessary. We imagine one reason so many men are considered bad patients is that they feel demeaned by their necessary dependency; being a patient is not very masculine. For your part, however close you are to him, even dependent on him, a nurse is tied to her patient and his needs in a way a wife will inevitably resent.

The opposite mistake is to become so overwhelmed by the impossibility of being prepared for your presumed role as all-in-one doctor, nurse, and heart monitor that you give up and do nothing at all, resigning yourself to despair and him to nervousness.

That is just as wrong. Because, in fact, there are a number of things you can and should do—all of them reasonably simple, none making you a nurse or your home any more a hospital auxilliary than it is right now.

Certain hospital-like arrangements would be perfectly normal in any home. When possible and appropriate, they should be made exactly that way: as things you might have done years ago, and probably should have done. (For instance, the emergency numbers on the phone, and the resuscitation training we shall describe in a moment.)

Other arrangements are strictly for the purpose of making sure your husband knows he will get help quickly if he needs it. They should be made frankly and openly, then ignored.

The first is about literally calling for help. Basically, that is what a heart monitor does. Incomparably sooner and faster than anything else can; but such speed is no longer necessary. Talk to your doctor about it with your husband. You will find out that even with the rare sort of massive coronary that is invariably fatal, there is time for the victim to call for help. (As a doctor pointed out to us, men are found in their cars, slumped over the wheel—but they had time to pull to the side of the road!)

So the only problem that can reasonably trouble even an advanced pessimist is: when he calls, will anyone hear?

First, you should make sure that for a week or so, someone will always be there to hear. Not a nurse. And not every second. But if you work, for example, or will be gone for several hours, arrange for someone to come in. A visitor, a mother's helper, someone to clean, to cook—anyone with normal hearing and normal intelligence. Do not ask your husband if he wants someone there. "Do you want me to get you a baby-sitter?" is how the question will come out, no matter how you phrase it. If you are hiring someone, tell your husband that (1) you need done whatever the person is ostensibly being hired to do and/or (2) you will not feel comfortable about leaving unless there is someone there in case he wants anything. It is for *your* peace of mind. He is supposed to be in bed; not hopping up and down to get a glass of juice or answer doorbells.

Even when you are at home, you will not be right there with him all the time. At least you shouldn't be! That's called "hovering" and is certainly anything but the normal home atmosphere to which he should be adjusting. Besides, both of you need some time to yourselves.

Still, for his sense of security, it is important that he be able to call you. Easily, without the strain of shouting. In an emergency, he might be unable to shout. Also (no small consideration), it will be hard for you to convince the children not to shout in the house if you and your husband have to shout every time he wants anything. And if "no shouting" was not already the rule in your home, it should be now; a heart patient should have a minimum of noise and turmoil.

Obviously, what you need is a call system.

It can be a fancy intercom system, wiring-in every room in your home. Or, less elaborately, his room and the one, two, or three rooms you are most likely to be in when you are not with him. Or, even more simply, the upstairs and downstairs or the front and rear of an apartment, split-level or ranch-style house. You can get an intercom system, with two stations, for under $10. And in a multistoried house, a large split-level, a sprawling or railroad apartment, it will be useful the rest of your life.

However, an intercom is a luxury, not at all a necessity, even for now.

The idea is to convince your husband that it will always be easy for him to summon aid. With that in mind, any sort of distinctive "call" is fine. A brass bell costing under a dollar has a loud, clear, and unmistakable urgency about it that makes it perfectly adequate. It should have a handle to which some sort of cord can be attached, with the other end tethered to a convenient part of the bed, keeping it always in reach, never knocked aside and inaccessible, under the bed or in a corner.

Whatever you decide upon, make sure it is in place before he gets home and can protest that no such thing is needed and you should not bother.

If any of his interests tie in with some sort of call system, by all means turn the call system into a "welcome home" gift. If he is a particularly keen hunter, for example, a new duck call can be the temporary call system (it should certainly be audible and distinctive enough!). Or a bicycle bell, if he happens to have joined the current movement toward bicycling.

One of the nicest systems we ever heard of was given by a Heart Wife in her mid twenties whose husband was an ardent sports car buff. His prize possession was a little English MG, the old model that looks like a miniature Rolls-Royce. He kept it in Swiss-clock running order and dazzlingly polished. She got him a huge, curlicued Bermuda taxi horn, which she shined up and mounted on the side of their bed, ready for service then, and later to be put on his car.

The only problem with any of these systems is that you may end up hating them all. Some Heart Wives get to feeling more and more smothered during the weeks that follow their husbands' homecoming. They are totally tied down and on call. They resent it deeply; and any call system, no matter how eventually useful or presently charming, quickly rankles as an overpowering symbol of how closed in and restricted their lives seem to them. We will examine this problem, later, in Chapter 15.

No matter how you finally feel about your local "call system," there cannot be two minds about the next step in the chain of getting help when it is needed.

A Heart Wife summed up the correct formula for arranging the second step:

> I found out where we could get help the fastest, then I pasted a label with the number right on the phone. I told the children this was the emergency number. Then I never mentioned it again.

If you have extensions, put the number on each one. If the emergency number is "O" for operator, find out what you should ask for, and add that to the sticker. Something like:

> EMERGENCY—Dial "Operator"
> Say: "Fire Department Rescue Squad"

You might also give the doctor's number. But that's *all*. In an emergency people are, by definition, rushed, excited, and frightened. So keep it simple.

If possible, ask your doctor about emergency calls and procedures when you are with your husband—who will get another message: the information and the knowledge that you are eager to take every element of risk out of his leaving the hospital.

Some arrangements lie between the areas of home and hospital. They make perfectly good sense, all on their own; but they obviously are inspired by your husband's needs. The most dramatic is the arrangement you should make to see that you and everyone else in your home knows the basic techniques of cardiorespiratory resuscitation.

One Heart Wife opened our eyes to the important effect this has on the other people involved, besides your husband. Actually, she might be called a "double" Heart Wife. Her first husband finally succumbed to multiple coronaries. After a while, she remarried. And not long ago her new husband had a mild attack—one that they both consider a warning to heed. Rigorously!

Here is how she describes the "hidden" advantage of knowing what to do until the ambulance gets there:

> Before my first husband had the pain that turned out to be the fatal coronary, we had all learned how to give heart resuscitation.
>
> I had gone to a YMCA class years earlier, in case we ever had an incident at our pool. And I discussed it with the boys at the time—you know, in case anybody ever needed it? Then they learned, too. And I think the fact that there was something we could do when my husband had the attack was very important. Because you panic. You think, "Now what do I do?" Well, we knew.
>
> One of the boys called the fire department. We administered heart massage; we gave mouth-to-mouth resuscitation.
>
> It didn't help. Nothing would have helped.
>
> But it was very important from the viewpoint of the boys that they knew how. They were there and they knew what to do and they knew they'd done everything anyone could have done.
>
> That was very important to how they felt about it. And they had done the right thing.

Important: Notice the order! *First* the call to the fire department—then everything else. Also notice they had *learned* how to administer aid. It is not difficult to learn; but it *must* be taught to you. It cannot be picked up by watching Dr. Welby do it on TV. Fred McCuiston, of the Los Angeles Fire Department Rescue Squad, told us that heart massage, especially, can be dangerous if improperly administered; in fact, only those members of the squad who have taken specific training are *permitted* to give cardiorespiratory resuscitation.

Call your local Y or the Red Cross or Heart Association or Police or Fire Department and find out about the nearest class. How many other things will you ever learn that can do considerable good even those few times when they do not help? Or are never even needed! Just knowing will boost your confidence. And your husband will surely appreciate the fact that you and the children have bothered to learn.

Another home-hospital compromise is a small, hand fire extinguisher. No home should be without one—ever. Certainly not your home, now. Why? In one of his books, former Secretary of State, Dean Acheson, said that one of the first things that struck him upon meeting President Franklin Roosevelt was the curious care with which the president, who had been crippled by polio as a young man, snubbed out each cigarette. It seemed almost obsessive. Then, suddenly, Mr. Acheson realized why. A person who is crippled and can't walk, much less run, out of a room in case of fire naturally takes considerable pains to make sure fires don't start anywhere near him.

Not that your husband is a cripple. But remember how unadvisable it is to expose him to heart-pounding excitement. What if a fire should break out? The least exciting way to handle it is with a small extinguisher. So put one right near the bed. Within a week or so it will not be necessary to keep it there; but it will still be something you certainly should have around the house.

There is one out-and-out hospital-like routine that you should follow without disguise: a written record of medication. Prepare a list of the exact medication and exact, day-by-day dosage required. Keep it unmovably near the medicine supply, with a pen or pencil firmly attached—and make it an inviolable rule to mark off medication as soon as it is taken from the bottle. Especially any "every four hours" or "after meals" medicines. One missed or one too many may not be the end of the world.

But it is worrisome; and there is no need for extra worry, especially when there is no reason for it.

Also keep separate at least a three-day supply of every medication your husband takes, rotating the supply with every fresh batch of medicine bought. That will help you avoid the otherwise inevitable Sunday evening scramble to find an open drugstore when you discover that someone miscounted or forgot and there is no more Coumadin or Dijoxin or whatever.

Better still, get from the nearest five-and-dime store a little plastic pill box with seven separate compartments, each marked with a day of the week. That way, the whole week's budget of medication is loaded in at one time and you always know when you are running out.

Finally, you might consider something that sounds like an unequivocal item of hospital supply—but actually has a very practical, even jolly, use. Oxygen! It is not very expensive. A small, but professional, inhalator costs about $20; refills run about $10, each. The point of refills is that if you never need it for your husband's heart, you may find it comes in handy for his head—or yours.

As Berton Roueché points out in his delightful and instructive book about alcohol, *The Neutral Spirit* (Little, 1960), pure oxygen is the best single relief known for a hangover. We mention it because the night *is* coming when you and your husband go out to celebrate the fifth or tenth or twenty-fifth anniversary of the day he came home! Boy Scouts think they are the only ones whose motto is "Be Prepared." They should see Heart Wives in action.

CHAPTER
12

Welcome Home, Stranger

The man who comes home is not the same man who went away. Neither physically nor mentally. In many ways he really is a stranger—and you must be prepared for some of the strangeness about him. Prepared by knowing what to expect and by being ready to help the stranger adjust to his home and his life.

Some of the ways in which he is different are constructive, and will be the foundation for good, solid adjustments later on, once the immediate problems of adjusting are out of the way. Not all the time a patient spends in the hospital is spent brooding, being hostile to his wife, and getting bored with daytime TV. A lot is spent thinking constructively. Many patients have told us this was the only chance they had in their adult lives, with time and motive both at hand, to take a close look at themselves and reevaluate where they are going in life. In the final analysis, what you have been doing up to this point is directed toward helping make that reevaluation, and the plans for the future that comes of it, healthy ones. What you do from now on has the same goal.

First, though, you have to get the stranger settled in. This chapter examines the problems you can expect to face doing it.

The changes start with the physical changes to his body

brought about by the time he has spent in the hospital, and his mind's reaction to those changes. The day he leaves the hospital he is convinced that this is a giant step forward.

Instead, it turns out to be a small step backward.

How come?

When the doctor tells your husband he is well enough, strong enough, recovered enough to go home, he means medically well, strong, and recovered. But home is charged with such emotional meaning, it equals "cured" and "recovered," whereas, in one area—physical strength—most patients are actually more worn out when they leave the hospital than when they went in.

The reason is called "atrophy," loss of muscle tone through inactivity. It happens to most any bed patients. And for heart patients, there simply is no way out: the heart must rest; which means the body must rest; which means (at first) immobility in the CCU, then gradual, slow, measured exercise in a regular hospital room. He gets all the exercise possible; but it is always well below the activity of normal living.

In terms of strength, you get out of a muscle exactly what you put in. The more you do, the more you can do. But the reverse is also true. The less you do in the way of exercise, the less a muscle can do. And the less it can do, the greater the exhaustion when strain is put on the muscle.

So there is your husband, his last day in the hospital, rested, relaxed, almost euphoric about how well his recovery is coming along. Why, he's going home! He is also debilitated and atrophied. Except he does not know that yet.

Then comes the first "violent" activity since the attack.

That is what going home amounts to for your husband. Getting up, getting dressed . . . *moving;* plus the excitement. Just "normal" activity; a little subnormal, if anything. But much more sustained, intense, and draining than any he has had for weeks.

When he suddenly finds out how weak he is, you know what that must do to his entire outlook. Your husband naturally translated his rested feeling into a feeling of strength. His mental attitude practically sported a sign, "Color me rosy." Finding out he was wrong can be a mental wipeout for him.

What can be worse than dashed hopes? What is more depressing? What kind of man gets tired from dressing and being driven home? What kind of man is unable to climb stairs, walk fast, or lift things (in fact, unable to do anything those first days at home but crawl into bed); why, no man at all—he tells himself.

You know how it goes. When you are depressed over anything, nothing looks half so promising as it did yesterday. You just sit and eat worms.

This is a terribly dangerous point in your husband's recovery. Not medically, of course. His physical condition did not change between the hospital and home, only his illusions about what that condition is. Some reaction to the disparity between how he felt upon leaving the hospital and how he feels when he steps —or shuffles—through the front door is certain. Maybe not quite despair, but surely sharp disappointment. Maybe not total pessimism, but surely a monumental case of "down in the dumps."

Since you know what is happening and why it is happening, you can help your husband understand.

Ask the doctor to warn him about how much weakness to expect and the reasons for it. The majority of doctors seem to restrict their warnings to what patients should *not* do: overexert themselves, lift things, climb stairs, and so on. You want your husband to know both what not to do—and what not to *think*. He must not think his hospital feeling of "every-day-in-every-way I'm getting stronger and stronger, better and better" had any more *real* physical basis than does his new, kitten-weak, baby-helpless feeling. Both are based on the plausible, but incorrect, premise that strength, vigor, and a rested feeling mean that his heart has healed—while a wretched, weak, tired feeling means his heart has not healed.

It just is not so.

By leaving the hospital, by "testing" his wonderful new

strength, your husband has put his unexercised and somewhat atrophied muscles through a draining exertion. But, far from either damaging his heart (or proving to himself that he had not really been making the progress he thought), he actually *was* taking a giant step—toward truly important strengthening of his heart. At the same time, he is strengthening his other muscles. Because his heart *must* have more exercise than it was getting while he was in the hospital. And the only way his heart can get exercise it needs is for the other parts of the body to be exercised.

If the consequences of how your husband feels were not apt to be unwholesome, the situation would be comical. Because the exact same physical reaction used to give him *pleasure,* a feeling of virtuous contentment!

Do you remember what happened when your husband would play the season's first round of golf or set of tennis, the first game of touch football or basketball since school (or after he finally got around to cleaning out the garage)? Any bout of unaccustomed and fairly strenuous exercise made him stiff, sore, and exhausted.

What is strenuous? To quote an old proverb (which we just now made up) "Strenuous is as strenuous has *not* been doing for a long while." And that means *anything* you have not been doing.

Before, it was merely a question of aching or sore muscles, a feeling easily equated by an otherwise healthy man with "getting back into shape." It is the signal for him to start concocting plans for "keeping it up" and "getting down to fighting weight." As the liniment goes on, the imagination takes off: is the exercise class at the Y enough, or should he see what a health club has to offer? How will his blue suit look with the shoulders and chest let out, the waist taken in? And whatever happened to that barbell set he got for his fourteenth birthday? In extreme cases, this condition has been known to last for the better part of a week.

The same—in reverse—goes for his present condition. Mostly

because of the difference in the level of activity. Before, he knew he was making unused muscles perform high deeds and did not find their protest unreasonable or frightening. This is different. How can simple, everyday actions tire and weaken any but a desperately sick and dangerously debilitated man?

Easily. It happens all the time. Literally—whenever any patient comes home from a few weeks in a hospital. And when the patient has been in the hospital with a coronary, there is added fear, apprehension, and a suggestion of more serious complications. But except for the possibility of some slight inefficiency in getting the blood pumped around the body, *the heart is not involved* in his weakness or tiredness.

If the doctor has explained this, your husband will surely feel less anxiety and less depression—and less resultant disappointment and anger.

Still, there are some general problems brought on by his weakness. What can happen? Well, there is a completely natural mistake you, the children, visitors—in fact, anyone around the home—will tend to make. You will instinctively want to "help" him do whatever appears "too much for him." We can tell you, flat out, that only one person is qualified to decide what is and what is not too much for your husband to do. The doctor. He will outline the limits of activity very clearly before your husband leaves the hospital. No one in your home should be permitted to "help" him do anything within those limits. There are two reasons. The first is to minimize the frequency, intensity, and number of what we call "Light Bulb Problems."

This is a category of problems you can expect to face in the early days of your husband's return—problems that come from his reaction to the trauma of his weakness. You must be aware of the stress, self-doubt, and anxiety that are bound to follow.

It is not enough to be hip to the dangers of "emasculation" and the more theatrical troubles of our psychiatrically sophisticated society. You can completely trip up on the *little* elements of friction. Then, when he reacts with the delicacy of a wounded water buffalo, it will be terribly hard to keep your post-Freudian cool. For example? We give you one from our own private stock of Things We Wish We Had Known—it is *why* we call these "Light Bulb Problems."

Two days out of the hospital, JoAnn's husband noticed a burned-out light bulb. Naturally enough, he decided to replace it. When he found that his hospital stay had left him too weak to even change a light bulb, he was sick with frustration. And all the more determined to *change that damned bulb.* Another fifteen minutes and Forrest had gone from being too weak to change a light bulb to even weaker, plus exhausted. At this point, enter JoAnn. She saw her husband sitting with new light bulb in hand (gathering strength for another assault; but how was she to know?), malevolently eyeing a burned-out bulb that, to him, seemed welded in place. Well, what kind of wife would hesitate a moment in such circumstances? (What kind? A smart one who had been warned about such things, that's what kind.) JoAnn sweetly took the bulb out of Forrest's hand and blithely started to change the bulb. The operation came to a sudden end as her husband exploded in anger and bitterness, bordering on rage.

Avoiding things like that would be reason enough not to "help" your husband do "simple, little things." His explosions of anger are not good for anyone's heart, his or the would-be "helper's." But the main reason is that his reaction, while neither pleasant nor good for his physical health (and absolutely horrible for everyone's mental health) is correct. His instinctive outburst is nature's way of saying, "Get lost, I need the exercise." In fact, within the doctor's limits, the harder something is to do, the more important it is for him to keep trying.

Two analogies make the situation clear; unfortunately it would be advanced folly to let on to him you are thinking of either one. Just between us, though, it is exactly like a baby learning to walk, or anyone who has suffered a sudden, crippling handicap relearning lost skills. You would never think of "helping" them. Far from being a kindness, it would be the most pitiless sort of meddling in a necessary and natural process, no matter how hard the "struggle" seemed to be.

That is exactly the case with your husband. His muscles must regain their tone; his heart must be exercised up to maximum strength, something that can be accomplished only by exercise that requires the heart to work harder than it does supplying the body's "at-rest" needs.

Another major problem of your husband's weakness concerns visitors. However, that problem gratifyingly diminishes in direct proportion to the amount of time that passes and the amount of exercise your husband gets during that time.

Taken all-in-all, visitors are welcome as the flowers of spring, even counting the odd thorn. They are an approximation of natural contacts with the normal world; they are a start toward adjustment. The only problem is that your husband may overdo it, seeing too many people too soon, staying up too late, getting tired, and not even in a constructive physical way, such as exercising and strengthening his muscles. Of course, exercising too much would also be bad; but that is less of a danger. Exercise is self-limiting. His body tires dramatically and tells your husband he has had enough.

Receiving visitors is different. It tires in a way that is not self-limiting and does not make your husband realize he has had enough and had better quit. What's more, the visitors may not be able to see that they are tiring him. Everyone is having such a good time!

You have to call a halt—because it is most unlikely your husband will, even if he feels "a little tired." How can he dismiss his visitors? Or admit that sitting and chatting with friends is too much for him. People are coming to "see how he is," aren't they? Well, by golly, he is going to show them! And he will scarcely want the demonstration to end with "Sorry, you'll have to run along, now; time for my nap." He will be less than enchanted to hear you say any such thing, either. So what do you do?

You do your own version of what this Heart Wife did:

> We started having visitors in at night, when he was still in bed. And he didn't know he was tired; anyway, he wouldn't admit it.

So, I would tell them beforehand, "Now, you're coming at eight o'clock, and I would be very happy if you would leave about ten. John is going to seem fine—and he is fine. But you know how he is: he'll get so excited seeing you! And we have to be careful." And they were perfectly marvelous! When the time came, they would say they had to go.

That should be all that is necessary. After all, friends are concerned about his health, too. When they know about the need for rest, most will want to do what is best for him; in fact, they will insist on doing it, even over his objections and his "Oh, I feel fine, don't run off yet!"

Still, there may be those who do not cooperate. If they forget what you have told them, hint. If that does not do it—well, do whatever it takes to shoo them away with as little embarrassment to your husband as possible. One Heart Wife covered both points when she told us:

> There were only one or two that were really very bad. What I generally did was insist that my husband be in bed while he had visitors. Because your body is more relaxed and at rest in bed.
> But mostly, *people get a message* when you're in bed!

We asked if she had ever been called upon to make the message a little clearer.

> Yes, sometimes. When I could see he was getting tired, I would say to them, "Well, it's been a grand visit! Now, come on, it's my turn for a visit with you!"

If the visitor is a real clod and simply cannot be managed, and you are pretty sure that anything more direct will simply provoke a scene, making your husband feel he must prove how well he is by insisting he is not a bit tired, you may decide that the extra fifteen minutes or half hour, or whatever, is not worth the hassle. All right, you will tell yourself, so this time he is not going to get quite the rest he should; he will be overtired. But that does not instantly result in a heart attack. In any long view, a scene is too high a price for a little extra rest.

But just wait until you get that clod of a visitor alone!

There is one more point to consider: should you serve visitors anything? Heart Wives seem to split between two points of view. And each is "correct." The answer depends entirely on how you and your husband feel about it. One view is:

> It's my nature to be a hostess. I would bring in coffee or tea.
> I didn't feel I had to entertain them, though. For me to make a pot of coffee was no trouble. And it was nice for my husband.
> It was important for him to feel that *he* was entertaining. I mean, he would want me to serve some coffee or tea to his friends and guests! What's the big deal?

If your husband feels the same, it is certainly an important factor. That same Heart Wife would agree, though, that if it takes on the proportions of "a big deal," the deal is off!

Other Heart Wives feel there are excellent reasons not to insinuate the slightest trace of "entertaining" into the visits. And they make a pretty strong case too:

> By serving cake or coffee, and making it a very social evening, visitors feel compelled, perhaps, to stay longer, or else they simply want to stay longer.
> You're talking about a sick man! You have a patient who's trying to get better. You want him to go to bed early. You don't want him to have to make long conversations or encourage visitors to stay on and on.

We asked the same Heart Wife how she handles what seems to be a very common problem that puts you in an unpleasant and ungracious position: when visitors bring him cake.

> I think you can handle it without being brusque or without being rude.
> The best thing is, you can say, "I would really prefer not to give him any. Thank you so much; but may we have it when the kids are around? It's really not good for him. He's trying to diet."
> I never for one minute thought, "Gee, they must have thought I was inhospitable for not having served anything." I figured if they're nice enough to want to come and visit, they should be able to understand that.

The consensus certainly is strongly against the slightest elaboration in entertaining visitors. What it comes down to is your evaluation of your own situation. If your husband will feel it is unforgivably inhospitable (perhaps chintzy) to not offer visitors some rudimentary refreshment, then fine. If you feel it is no bother, fine. But we urge you to fix in mind the distinction between these visits and any form of "social occasion." They are social only by the loosest of definitions. Really, they are therapy—as totally a part of your husband's recovery and adjustment as his medicine and his exercises. The more lighthearted aspects of having visitors must not be allowed to get in the way of your husband's rest or diet. Or of your efficiency. Or the closeness of your relationship with your husband.

This last consideration should be the keynote of any activities you can arrange for him during the early stages—that is, while he is still spending most of his time either actually in bed or at least around home.

Anything you can do together should be given first priority.

If it is an activity that evokes some pleasant projection of the future, all the better.

If he started some learning project while in the hospital, you may be able to help him, if only as "quizmaster" when he is reviewing each lesson.

One excellent activity that is much better done by two than by one is learning a language. If both of you like travel and it seems at all likely you may be able to do some, and if you have always thought about taking a trip to a foreign country, this is a fine time to learn the language. You can get a set of language course records for about $10.

And for "a donation" (which means whatever you want to give), you can join the International Association for Medical Assistance to Travelers. The main feature of membership is a booklet listing English-speaking doctors in every major city around the world, all of whom have agreed to a charge of $8 for an office visit. The address of the association is 350 Fifth Avenue, New York, New York 10001.

Even if you are unlikely, unwilling, or unable to go out of the country on your next vacation, or if the only country you really want to see is England, even then, your husband might get interested in really *planning* a trip. Routes, sights, accommodations—the works. A few letters to oil companies, chambers of commerce, and state historical societies will bring a flood of free planning material.

And speaking of letters, now is the time for him to answer all cards, letters, and phone calls asking after his health. It is something that you can do together very nicely; and the chances are he will be glad to have your services as a secretary.

We emphasize the "togetherness" in these activities, because that is a good offset, if not antidote, for the next problem that can come up to poison the air—and your relationship.

You Are the Enemy

"Now, really!" we hear you say at this point, "is there no end to it?"

Hostility was one thing when he was still in the hospital, understandably shaken by the attack, scared and uncertain about the future, mad at fate and the world for the dirty trick played on him, and with only you to kick back at. But now?

Now there seems to be no personality change. It is the real him; and the real him must hate the real you, because he is chronically angry and hostile, with a low, smoldering, and altogether convincing anger.

This time his bouts of anger and hostility are not apt to be detached from real causes, either. That was another easier-to-take feature of his in-hospital hostility. No one likes to be a target; but when we are, for clearly no cause, the bewildered resentment we feel is our solace. We have no feeling that maybe it was something we did. Now that has all changed. Certainly his anger and hostility are out of all proportion to whatever "offense" sets them off, but they are responsive to real events. It is as though you were dealing with a bundle of raw nerve endings. Anything can trigger an explosion. Merely the hint of being rubbed or crossed. Go about your business normally, and he explodes. "How can a man get any rest with a constant hullabaloo going on!" Walk on tiptoes over fragile eggshells, and he explodes. "How can a man relax with everyone sneaking around the place all the time!" Try what you will, it doesn't matter. Nothing you do is right. Nothing pleases; everything annoys and infuriates.

Nearly the only element of his hostility that makes it at all easier to take than it was before is the fact that you get to "share" it. No one seems immune. Offsetting that is the fact that this time his hostility may last a lot longer. Months, in extreme cases.

Is there, indeed, no end?

Of course there is. But at times it will seem as though you are going to have to take that on faith. There will not be much evidence.

Why should it be happening now? He is making good progress, getting stronger every day; before long he may be back to work. So why now? He got over his hostility, or seemed to. Why again?

Then the thought strikes: is it you? The way you are treating him? Are you being too driving? Too indulgent? Are you pushing him? Smothering him? Is it your fault, after all?

Probably not. In fact, one good index of how well you are doing your part in his recovery while he is home is his building, low-grade anger and his hostility. That does not seem like much of a "reward" for doing things the way you should; but the real reward, once this passes, is a better, closer life and a firmer adjustment to a new way of life for both of you. And for the rest of the family.

Here's why.

Start with his anger, and keep in mind your husband's position at this point in his life as you ponder these words by Dr. Kenneth House, a psychiatrist who has done much work with heart patients:

> In order to teach our children self-sufficiency, we teach them

to give up their natural desires to be dependent, to be loved and taken care of by others. We teach them to be more on their own and less "coming to Mommy and Daddy."

So little children often develop fantasies that if they are in a helpless, dependent position, they may be harmed—monsters may get them, or whatever.

As we grow up, part of us strives to stay away from this dependency and strive toward self-sufficiency. However, deep down, each of us knows dependency means love—tender, loving care and so forth. It's perfectly normal—yet we deny this to ourselves. And this creates in us frustration, and also a chronic state of anger . . . that we're not getting the dependency-care human beings want and really need.

Either way you lose.

If he lets himself go, lets himself sink into the "comfort" of dependency, he can become a "cardiac cripple." He is having some doubts about masculinity, anyway: remember what the doctor/patient said in Chapter 10 about the terrible feelings of castration typical of a heart patient. It would be easy enough for him to become dependent, given his state of mind and the physical facts of his recovery. He *is* more dependent than he has ever been in his adult life. And on whom? You, primarily. The other family members next. Realizing that, it takes no deep psychological insight to see where his anger will be directed.

At the same time, he is fighting dependency. That is natural and healthy, since it means he is struggling *not* to be a cardiac cripple. But as Dr. House points out, repressing his desires for dependency creates more anger. And it is directed at those on whom we would like to be dependent—those who, by the twist of the emotion's "logic" we all experience, are "denying" him their support.

No, it doesn't make "sense"; but you know how it feels. We all do the same thing. In effect, we blame others for not being perfect, for not being able to resolve for us the paradox of wanting something and not accepting it because we know we must not allow ourselves to have it.

There is another, more straightforward reason for his anger

and disappointment at this stage of recovery. It is implicit in
"The Light Bulb Problem." As he struggles and works to
regain his strength, it is evident to him that he does not seem as
fit and restored as he was in the hospital. And if he does not feel
stronger, how can he be getting stronger? (If you have ever
gone to an exercise class, you know the feeling: you can do less
the second visit than you could on the first.) You can see how
this must appear to your husband like a distinct reversal of
progress. He does not notice his improvement; he just notices
how tired he gets and how easily, which makes drooping spirits
all but a certainty and a returning of anger more than likely.

We suspect that there may be still another reason for you
being the target for that anger. After all, he came home to *you*.
And look! he's helpless, weak as a kitten—all (aha!) on *your*
account!

COUNTERATTACK

You have three choices for coping with his hostility at this point:

RETALIATE!: Fight back, give as good as you get. Why put
up with senseless attacks and general (there just is not any other
way to describe it) bitchiness from a grown man who has been
given no cause for his sudden temper? Give him hell!

IGNORE IT: Simply pretend you do not hear him. Close your
ears to his nastiness, close your eyes to his meanness. Why make
trouble?

DO SOMETHING: Take some corrective action that does
not involve either a retaliation or pretending his hostility does
not exist.

The first two methods have something to be said for them. So
we will say it: they are wrong. And wrong specifically because
they are tempting.

The first is satisfying: nothing is more so than hitting back at
someone who not only hit first, but who is clearly in the wrong.

The second has the attractiveness of martyrdom. The only

thing you need is a bland smile—and teeth strong enough to be clenched almost continually for a month or so.

It would be hard to say which is a more effective way to drive your husband up the wall. It depends on your personality and his. In any case, both retaliation and ignoring achieve the same "result": they keep the old fire raging, they put bounce and vigor into what could peter out as an argument. They are equally bad.

The third is a mixture of the first two. And it is the hardest—just as the hardest part of a recipe is that little phrase "Adjust the seasoning." Suddenly we are out of the realm of fixed instructions and thrown sharply on our own evaluations and our own concoction of remedies for things that have gone inexplicably "off," no matter how faithfully we have followed instructions up to that point. We do not blame Marion or Julia or Craig. They cannot tell what the conditions are in our kitchen, how heavy or light a hand we use in measuring. We hope you do not blame us: you will have to adjust your response in each circumstance, guided by your own sense of what is needed.

However, we can give you a good idea of the ingredients you will need at hand. Or let a Heart Wife tell you:

> I have to be better-natured, more understanding of the times when he reacts. But no matter what I tell myself, I'm still human, and there are still going to be . . . *times!*

There you have it: good nature, patience, love, perception, and understanding. And the greatest of these, for this situation at least, is understanding. Not just of him and why he is angry and hostile right now, but also of yourself—of any human being, really. The same Heart Wife went on to say:

> There are times when I feel that he's . . . "flexing his muscles" a little bit, and I hope to be in a mood to be sensitive, to be wise enough to know this is simply that kind of expression. I don't always know. Sometimes I react, and I don't always remember that he's sick.

I'm very sensitive. And when somebody's harsh with me, I don't like it. And if he's harsh with me out of his own needs, and I forget momentarily what's causing it—you know, it's like any relationship: I may snap back. We may have words.

You may, too. But then, you "had words" from time to time, before the heart attack. Well, that is simply another aspect of the normal life and relationship to which both of you must get reaccustomed. It is why making proper adjustments to the "seasoning" of your relationship is such a delicate, personal matter.

You must have patience, but so must he. When he is unfair and unjust, you are not doing him any good when you habitually ignore it. You have feelings, too. And if you understand yourself and your emotional needs, you can lovingly tell him just that. He is being unreasonable and hurting you and you are not happy about it.

You can take two positive actions that will, in a sense, control his hostility. Here is the first "battle plan" in the only kind of counterattack that makes sense for you. It is straight from a master strategist:

> I tried going out during the day when our two daughters were off at school. I hated leaving him alone, but it seemed to work. He had time to gather his thoughts and kind of compare being alone and having us there.
>
> And, of course, I kept hitting the fact that he really was getting stronger all the time. That helped. But mostly, I think, it was just letting him have some time to himself, so he didn't feel surrounded—and maybe he could even start to feel that he missed us.

And here is the second, also in the strategist's own words:

> We were very lucky in that we have very many wonderful friends—and there wasn't a day that somebody didn't come over to visit him.
>
> And it happened that with two couples the women were on a trip and the men were alone. Well, I had them here almost every night! Because when they were there, my husband was fine! [laughing] He only complained—and was miserable—around us!

Those are the two weapons of incalculable power in your arsenal:

GET OUT: Give him some time alone, some time to miss you and talk sense to himself. (It is more effective coming from him to himself anyway.)

BRING PEOPLE IN: Make sure there are fairly regular visitors. Let him look forward to seeing new faces.

As a side benefit, both plans give you a sort of furlough from your role as Heart Wife, helping you avoid the enervation and stiffled feeling that makes it so much harder to keep control of yourself and of situations as they come up.

Bringing people in is even more essential—as many visitors as your husband's strength (and doctor) will allow. For all we said about the potential problems of limiting visiting hours in the last chapter, remember that we also said visitors were therapeutic. Besides spelling you (no small value in itself), your husband gets a furlough from his role as patient—and grouch. And he needs that respite as much as you, maybe more!

One Heart Wife summed up the whole period of at-home hostility when we asked her if she could think of anything beneficial that came out of it:

Well, the only thing I got out of it I'm really glad about is . . . *me!*

You will get out of it, too. It will end. And all the sooner, the better you do your job.

CHAPTER

13

The Children: Now and Forever

You always knew you were going to have problems with your children. Not because of the heart attack. All that does is change a few of the forms the problems take. As we look at some of those forms, keep in mind that nothing has really changed: you have children; your children have problems and give you some—you knew they would when you had them—and you decided the problems were well worth the rewards. We are going to examine the immediate problems you may have with them, those you might have as soon as your husband gets home. What you do will diminish the number of problems you will have with your children (because of the heart attack, that is) in the future. This chapter is for now—and forever.

Start with what a Heart Wife told us about her daughters' part in their father's early recovery—and why she had them play that part:

> The first couple of weeks he had to have all his meals in bed. And I felt it was very important that the children be made a part of helping take care of him. My girls are great nurses: they would bring the trays and they would help him brush his teeth—not that he was an invalid, or anything—but they enjoyed it, and it made them feel needed. That was the most important thing the children really needed—to *feel* needed.

That's what children are all about! They need to be needed.

They need to be loved—and to be reassured that they are loved and needed.

Pretend it is some months ago, before your husband's heart attack; pretend you have just overheard someone saying the same thing—except that you missed the first part of what she said and managed to hear only this much: ". . . but they enjoyed it and it made them feel needed . . . etc." Would you instantly recognize her as a Heart Wife? Hardly. Her words make good sense coming from any parent talking about the general emotional needs of children under any circumstances.

Then what is there about the fact of a heart attack that makes those words seem so much to the point?

To start with, they remind you that what you know as a parent is not suddenly obsolete because you are, now, also a Heart Wife. Sometimes the Heart Wife in you will have to overrule the parent. About noise, for instance. Making noise ranks somewhere between an inalienable right and a sacred duty in most children's minds. So, as a parent, you probably feel that, as a rule, a certain amount of racket is no great sin against nature, or even household decorum. But, as a Heart Wife, you know their father's need for rest may make you forbid even a normal hullabaloo, especially during the first weeks after his return from the hospital. It does not mean your judgment as a mother is wrong, just that it has been temporarily displaced by circumstance. It is simply a matter of priorities.

Setting those priorities would not be terribly difficult—for a computer. That description, however, fits a rather small number of Heart Wives. The medical implications of your husband's needs can easily overwhelm you. You can be intimidated by the possible consequences of "anything going wrong," and soon lose all perspective on anything that may affect your husband's health and recovery.

Besides, there is the sheer novelty of your role as a Heart Wife. You have been a parent longer; you take that function in stride. You have not gotten the hang of being a Heart Wife, so everything connected with that role is strange and momentous.

As a result, you may overestimate the importance of what you do as a Heart Wife compared to what you do as a mother.

Even when your children's problems bear no discernible relationship to your husband's heart attack, you may start to judge them in terms of the heart attack. In that light, of course, they can seem laughably trivial. In which case you may dismiss them as not needing attention, unless they might conceivably interfere with a solution to . . . The Problem. Then the only "solution" is to forbid the problems. In everyday situations this translates as something on the order of "No, you may not try out for the football team—it would upset your father not to be able to go to the games to watch you, or your studies might suffer and low marks might worry your father, or you might get hurt and that would *kill* your father!" Or, "No, you may not go out on a movie date—your father would worry too much." Or, "No, you may not complain about the creepy way your [choose the appropriate one] big/little/twin sister/brother is behaving; your father is disturbed when he hears you fight." What you are really saying—to yourself—is that your children do not really have problems, that no one does, really. Except your husband.

That way of thinking is bad enough in its effect on you. If it communicates itself to the children—depending on how they take such things—the notion that any problem of less than cardiac dimensions is no problem at all can have an outcome that approaches tragedy. And it is all the more tragic for the complete absence of a villain.

For instance, a Heart Wife we shall call "Mrs. X" was thoroughly sensible about nearly all the things she did during her husband's early recovery period. But she did tell us that she felt her own problems, worries, and needs had to be almost totally repressed, for fear they might affect her husband. We have no reason to believe she foisted that view on her children; there was no sign of it in her two daughters, anyway. But somehow, with her son, who was away at a summer camp at the time of the heart attack, things were different.

MRS. X: Before the attack he was very close to his father. They would go camping with the Boy Scouts, everything! They had a great relationship. And I was worried about what was going to happen.

H.W.C.: How did your son react?

MRS. X: Well, he was extremely upset. He called me and he wanted to come home, and I said, "No." I thought it was better that he stay. There was nothing he could do.

So he stayed at camp until my husband came home. From that point on their whole relationship was different. He was terrified that if he upset his father in any way, he might cause him to have another heart attack.

Seeing that look on his face—years later, when his father would come home at night, and the first thing he'd say was, "How do you feel?"—it's so wrong!

H.W.C.: How did you feel about it at the time?

MRS. X: I really felt very unhappy for him because I realized that it wasn't a normal growing-up situation. He was always very, very careful not to anger his father; always to do what he thought would make his father happy.

H.W.C.: How old is he now?

MRS. X: He's twenty-five.

H.W.C.: Does he ever talk about it?

MRS. X: No, he doesn't. Although we have discussed the fact that he was overly careful about his attitudes and how he treated his father. And he thought, before he did anything, just what the reaction might be to his father and if it might endanger his health. And that's not very wholesome.

H.W.C.: Did you realize it at the time?

MRS. X: Well, in retrospect, I guess I partly realized it then. But I didn't think, then, that I should do anything. I felt it would be more detrimental to my husband to make it an issue then.

And I felt, "Well, too bad about the relationship

between father and son, but it's something I think that
he'll have to get over." But I don't think he ever did get
over it.

Who is to blame? The husband for not knowing something
was wrong? The boy for his tippy-toe reaction? The mother for
her decision that a man with a heart attack needs a considerate
son more than a teen-age boy needs a hiking companion? To ask
the question—that way, at least—is to answer it. No one is to
blame. But *some thing* is! The word "need."

For all the reasons we have mentioned, a Heart Wife often
mentally demotes her children's needs to *wants*. After all, her
husband is the one who is sick, not her children. What do they
really need? The answer is they need what they have always
needed, your love and attention. They simply cannot have all
the love and attention they want—or even need—all of the time.
It is a matter of setting sensible priorities, and sensibly adjusting
them to match changing circumstances. It does not mean ignoring the children or their needs. See how sensibly it can work
out: here is what a Heart Wife told us about how she handled
the problem of her children's need for her while she spent
nearly a solid month with her husband, who had a total of three
coronary incidents before he was released from the Coronary
Care Unit. We asked her if she had felt any guilt about leaving
the children to themselves so much:

> I suppose I felt guilty now and again, but I didn't have time to
> indulge myself with guilt.
> I mean, so they were going to suffer a little bit! It was much
> more important that I be with him. But I guess I should say that
> I was always there, with them for dinner. I would feed him at the
> hospital—what is it, a five-o'clock feeding? Then I'd run home
> and feed the kids at six.
> I was too keyed up to eat. But I would sit and have a salad or
> something. The thing that mattered was I was there with them.

Certainly she had to overrule what she knew as a
mother—that, in fact, children do need their mother and do

"suffer" without her. But between two competing needs, she had to choose the one that was literally life-and-death. That was top priority. And *then* she took care of priority number two.

When her husband was better, the balance of her time at home and at the hospital changed. The priorities changed to suit the circumstances.

If you continue to see your children's needs as valid claims even when you must subordinate them to the more urgent needs of a heart patient, you will almost automatically arrange to do it without making the children ever feel they are any less loved and needed. Not by you, not by their father.

Of course, your children will continue to have problems—the same ones they had before the attack, and would have had if there was no heart attack. But there really is nothing special about these normal, growing-up problems. They are no more serious (but, alas, no less serious) than before. If you are satisfied that you generally handle them pretty well, keep doing whatever you have always done. Problems that have no connection with the heart attack should be kept that way. The ones that do have a connection come up often enough, and are more than troublesome enough, so that you need none added to them.

Problems related to the heart attack come in different shapes and sizes. But they have the same origin. And, in reality, they are not *special* heart-attack problems at all; instead, they are ordinary problems magnified by the heart attack. And they all come back to the basic need of your children to feel needed, wanted, and loved. Specifically by you.

Neither of us has any formal training in psychiatry. But it is not necessary to burrow deep into Freud or to rattle off terms like Oedipus and Electra complexes to pinpoint the main problem area—one that did not start with their father's heart attack but is blown up out of all proportion by your necessary reaction to the heart attack.

Long before Freud, parents realized that as they shared each other with the children, the children had to share each parent with the other. Of course, very small children want *all* of whatever they want. In a way, learning to share and growing up are synonymous.

Usually that is more or less all right. They do have a lot of you. But after the heart attack, they have less of you: less of your time, less attention, less sheer physical presence most likely. Much less when your husband was in the hospital; but they will continue to have less than usual, even now, when your husband is home. And in the future as well. Certainly, your children will continue to have noticeably less of your absorption in them and their affairs. And that will be true for a number of years to come. Perhaps forever. So it is important that they realize that your interest in them and your love for them have not changed—just your absorption. You have their father's health on your mind.

Your shift of absorption and your necessary reordering of priorities may mean that your children will feel themselves somewhat dispossessed. What was theirs will be, in some degree, less theirs. And the evidence is all around them.

It will not be quite *their* home anymore. Especially not at first—which is precisely when they will feel the strangest about the whole situation, anyway. There definitely will be a need for a lot more quiet than there ever was before. They cannot have their friends trooping in at any hour (if at all).

It is not quite *their* father, either. Again, especially at first. Suddenly Little League is not quite so important as it seemed. There might be an empty seat at the father-son banquet. In fact, there will be a total absence of the more robust father-son activities at first, and "any at all" will take considerable working up to. "Daddy's little girl" is not going to get swept up for a big squeeze and a kiss, not for a terribly long time.

If they are too young to have visited him in the hospital, even the way he looks may have changed. And they will never have seen him looking . . . weak! Remember, this is their father, their protection against the world. "My ol' man c'n lick your ol' man" may not be a line actually used outside of cartoons, but there is palpable truth in what it says about how children tend to think of their fathers. Now suddenly here is a wraith who cannot even walk up a flight of stairs. It can be pretty frightening.

Naturally, all these things are felt less acutely by older children. But the central problem of feeling dispossessed is common to children at any age. The sophistication that helps older children understand the physical aspects of their father's heart attack merely means they are in for reactions that are more sophisticated, not less unpleasant.

Parents can flatter themselves that they have not only their children's love, but their friendship, that they are their children's pals. Maybe so. But they are also authorities, providers, supervisors, and—an often overlooked, but highly important function of parents for their children—an audience and cheering section. No parent who was ever given a report card to sign, good or bad, can doubt it. There is an immense need on the part of children, at almost any age, to feel they have the interested attention of their parents. Approval, too, undoubtedly; but all we are talking about, here, is attention—measured in time, eagerness to hear, and absorption. It is a rude blow to children when they discover their parents have any *other* interests in the world besides them.

With this in mind, review the situation as it must appear to your children.

While he's in the hospital, chances are they'll have to get along without you some of the time—and probably not get your full attention, even when you're with them; when he gets home, you will seem even more preoccupied at first. Which means they're going to be missing a full-time father, for a period of weeks, and have, at best, a part-time mother for months to come. Unlike the effect of his altered appearance, which will really affect only the younger children, his virtual disappearance as an effective father—and maybe more important, his monopolization (intentional or not) of their mother's time and attention—can affect children of any age.

The result can be devastating on children—again, at any age. For example, we offer this transcript of our notes after our first

in-hospital meeting with a Heart Wife who was seeing her
husband through a second attack some four years after his first:

> When he had his first attack, his son was fifteen years old. Not
> long after he came home from the hospital, the son began to
> exhibit symptoms of a heart attack, too.
> They got more and more severe, until the boy simply
> couldn't function. He was put through every conceivable EKG
> and enzyme test—all negative. There simply was no heart in-
> volvement, at least not in a cardiac sense. He then started to
> receive psychiatric help, and it soon became clear that his
> mother's almost total attention to her husband's health had made
> the boy terribly jealous, and his subconscious mind conspired
> with his body to produce the thing that his emotions recognized
> as the most "effective" way to get attention: a heart attack. Just
> like dear ol' Dad's, the one that gets all of Mom's attention.

The adjustment that you and your husband make to each
other and to the life-style necessary for successful survival in the
years to come must include your children. And their feelings of
dispossession at this point in recovery can create havoc, even if
it is not so noticeably dramatic.

The resolution of this case can point the way around the
problem for you. There was an instance of "neglect." We do
not mean to suggest that any observer would have felt that the
Heart Wife was neglecting her son. But this side of complete
unreality, neglect is in the heart of the slighted. Uncontestably,
the fifteen-year-old boy felt he had a slighting amount of attention, necessarily less than he was used to. And that is what
your children, of any age, will receive—automatically, because
you *must* spend less time with them, mentally and emotionally,
even if you somehow manage not to spend less time physically.
There is no choice. It is not humanly possible for your emotional energy, or even simple attention, to be riveted on them
and their lives. Not for some time to come. And they are bound
to know it.

So there is no "cure" for their feeling dispossessed; they are
not imagining it; you really are less involved with them, less

caught up by what they do, what they say, and what they feel. Their father's usurpation of the central place in your arrangement and management of your home is real—and necessary.

But there is an antidote for any extreme reaction.

In the case of the fifteen-year-old, the psychiatrist dug out the feelings of neglect that so bothered the boy; and he helped him understand that his mother's sudden shift of "interest" from him to his father had nothing to do with love but with a real physical need on his father's part. Incredibly, no one had explained to the boy exactly what was involved in recovery from a heart attack, what the need for rest was, or exactly how any woman can be expected to react to the danger involved in a heart attack. No one had bothered to help the boy think through what any human being in his mother's position *must* be feeling and fearing, or what the sure results of those emotions must be.

When he did know, the boy had little trouble grasping the fact that his mother did not love him less, but that she was reacting, herself, to an immediate and important need that his father had.

The way to avoid any such reactions in your children is to do for your children what the psychiatrist had to do: make them aware that

— their father has needs right now, physically and emotionally, that will demand a larger portion of your time and energy;

— an apparent shift in your "interest" from them to their father is a direct result of the physical/medical facts of their father's heart attack and of your own need at this point;

— the rearrangements, dislocations and reorientations of the household, their dispossession, your "neglect"—none of these has a thing to do with your love for them; it is possible to love different people in different ways and be wholehearted, but not possible to concentrate on two different people, any more than it is physically possible to think two thoughts or say two words, both at the same time;

— when they were babies, their needs came first—with both you
and their father; now, because of the same physical situation
(one party being able to fend for himself, the other not), his
needs must come first.

Then all you do is add the usual amount of love, the usual
amount of interest and concern in them and their affairs that you
usually do—whenever you are with them.

And remember, they *are* children. That has two important
meanings in this instance, both of which work in your favor. If
they are literally children, in their very early teens or younger,
they have the amazing resiliency of youth. One Heart Wife
expressed it perfectly, adding another important point:

> They were awfully happy to see him. They made a "Wel-
> come Home" sign and they had stuff like that all over the place.
> They did it themselves; this was all on their own—they were so
> excited. But within two days it was as though he had never left.
> As you know, children return very rapidly. And I had talked
> to them, as much as I could, about "Now, we are going to have
> to take it easy; we can't have screaming and door-slamming
> every five minutes." And kids understand a helluva lot more
> than we think they do.

They do "return" with unbelievable rapidity, which gives
you tremendous leeway for slight tactical errors in how you
handle things.

If the children are older, especially if they are going through
puberty, the stresses are greater, the effect of fancied slights
more potentially serious. But the understanding is proportion-
ately greater, too.

Besides they are *your* children—at any age; there is the bond
of blood and affection that makes allowance for faults and
overrides even conclusive evidence of frailty on either side. So
with a reasonable explanation, suiting the language and
complexity to the age of the children, you should avoid anything
even approaching true upset.

For all the love and abiding concern you do have for your
children—including concern over their possible misapprehen-

sion of the shifted focus of your intense concern—there is no help for it. You must make that shift. There are times when your positive duty as a Heart Wife must take precedence over your inclinations as a mother—even if it means circumventing your husband's inclinations as a father. For example, again using the level of commotion you allow your children to make, you cannot afford to let your husband be put in a position where he may be tempted to say, "Oh, that's all right, kids, I wasn't *really* sleeping." It is *not* all right; and he cannot safely indulge the children, at first. Again it is a matter of establishing priorities. And setting rules that reflect the priorities. What they are, specifically, depends on your assessment of the situation and on your children. One Heart Wife we talked to was gratified by her children's cooperation:

> They were perfectly marvelous. And the parents on the block were marvelous, too. They were always inviting them to their houses.
> Or I would allow one of my kids to have one friend in.
> Next day, another of the children could have one friend in. But the kids were very nice about the whole thing.

When we asked another Heart Wife her reaction to that plan, she replied:

> My children brought no one in—at all. Not for, oh—it was a couple of weeks, three or four. You know, until he got used to being back at home. Out of the hospital, and even out of bed. It takes getting used to. And a lot of sleep and rest.
> It wasn't necessary for him to hear the noise and the excitement. Because you can't ask kids just to sit and not make noise. They're bound to.
> It would be an aggravation, hearing all that. And he couldn't even get up and go to another room. Either he'd have to shout and say, "Quiet"—then he feels mean—or he'd have to lie there and take it, not sleeping or resting.

It is not a matter of the first set of children being cooperative and the second set, not. But different children—and different fathers—have different hang-ups. So why strain what will surely be your children's desire to help?

That is generally what children do want. Fact is, we regularly run across astounding instances of children totally understanding what is expected of them.

But you must actively *give* yours a chance—which means giving them the information they need to understand what is expected of them, and why. It does not matter how old they are. Children of any age must have certain things about their father's condition explained to them. At a bare minimum, you owe your children—and your husband—two kinds of explanations.

First, they should understand the possibility that their father may seem . . . well, select a word appropriate to the age and understanding of the children. Call him cranky, hostile, upset, fringe-paranoid, whatever—but *tell* them ahead of time what to expect and (more or less) why, so they don't think their father has gone bananas, or suddenly hates them. Or, worst of all, holds them responsible for the attack.

Just as important, they must understand enough about their father's physical condition so they recognize the consequences of deliberate misbehavior—which children *are* capable of when provoked. Face it, children who normally are of such a sweet temper as might shame the angels still have lurking in them some of the more survival-oriented qualities of wild animals. They attack when hurt; they know exactly where the jugular is and how to go for it with awesome accuracy. The child has not been born who does not know precisely the words to say and the things to do that will infallibly drive parents up the wall.

It may be a comic-strip cliché to have funny old Daddy gone all purple in the face and practically foaming with rage over some Katzenjammer Kids antics. But the real-life consequences are no joke. Not now.

You know if it is apt to happen. If there is liable to be tension, a problem, whatever. If so, and if you cannot honestly tell yourself that a serious talk ahead of time will defuse any potential explosion, you must make some sort of arrangement to bypass the problem. Even if it means doing something that, under other circumstances would be totally unadvisable, like sending the children off somewhere for the first month or so of your husband's at-home recuperation. That would be extreme. But it is better all around, almost imperative—and as much or more for your children's sake than for your husband's. All "funny old Daddy" has to do is keel over while being infuriated by the children, and you will get a first-hand view of what guilt is all about.

Of course, intentional misbehavior is unlikely. Much more usual is the by-product of interfamily squabbles, ranging from annoyance, up. What can you do about it? There are two schools of thought among Heart Wives we have talked with. The first (quoting from notes we took during a post-hospital Heart Wife meeting) was:

> When the children had problems that she felt might possibly put a burden or strain on her husband, Mrs. X assumed the role of total buffer and peacemaker, making it very clear to the children that they in no way were to disturb their father. Not with problems, not with raised voices.
>
> Anything that had to be handled—as problems with teenagers must be handled—would have to go through her. And, although she did not appear to welcome the role, she felt it was necessary for her husband's welfare.

The other viewpoint was put vehemently by another Heart Wife:

> This is how you affect the children! Because you warn them: "Verboten! Don't get him upset. Tell me about it, don't tell him about it!" I don't think this is too good for the children. I think it has an effect on them. Maybe a permanent effect.

We tend to agree with the second viewpoint. But it is certainly a decision that is most properly based on your own style of raising your children and running your home, on their personalities, on yours, and on your husband's. Our only qualm is that such a specific short circuit of household routine, on such a

.delicate point, may tend to embellish "not bothering daddy" with dread, rather than consideration. By taking consideration for their father out of the realm of self-control and putting it into an under-no-circumstance-will-you class, you might so inhibit any normal response in your children to the stresses of normal living that they will overreact to the situation and magnify the need for restraint and caution in dealing with their father out of all proportion.

Your husband needs quiet; he needs rest. But it is not all-or-nothing. One disturbed sleep, one hour less of rest, one upset, one tumult (with or without shouting)—or two or three, for that matter, or any or all—these are not the end of the world. Or of him. If your children steal an hour's sleep from their father, it is barely petty larceny, and no one's best interest is served by turning it into a "federal case."

Besides, the most effective technique is not to exact compliance, but to get the children on your side, which is where their natural sentiment and affections encourage them to be, anyway. By angling your discussion toward the idea "Here's what you can do to help Daddy get better," you make them part of his recovery—and proud of the part. Daddy's going to be pretty proud, too, which is not a bad bonus. It is also a dandy way to get them to do what you want them to do.

The only problem is our natural tendency to think that only positive ways of helping can give children a graphic demonstration of how they are quite literally needed. But there are more instances in which the most cooperative thing a child can do is nothing. That gets sticky. It is very difficult to con children into believing that doing nothing is anything but nothing. *Not* making noise, *not* disturbing their father, *not* complaining about lack of attention or participation by you and your husband in their affairs, *not* goading Daddy into unwise activities—none of these has the attraction of positive action for anyone, least of all children. Yet they are essential for a smooth recovery. What can you do about it?

Well, you cannot hope to have children approach forbearance with the same zeal as they do positive ways of helping their father's recovery. But you do have their tremendous need to feel helpful working for you. The need to feel they have done something, made a significant contribution, is perhaps the strongest long-term emotion children have in connection with their father's heart attack.

When one Heart Wife's husband was stricken, he was water-skiing with his children. His teen-age daughter and early-teen son performed with unbelievable coolness. His youngest son, then age eight, was also in the boat. Later, the Heart Wife was proudly telling friends what Susie and Pete had done. When she paused for the totally justified applause to start, the youngest spoke up. "I helped, too," said Jimmy. "I didn't ask any questions."

On reflection, he may just have displayed the most astounding "cool," the most dumbfounding restraint, of all three.

One way to convince children that doing "nothing" is important is to turn it around and make something of nothing. Present them with a course of action that at least appears positive. For example, one Heart Wife had accompanied her husband on a business trip, and he had his heart attack very far away. She felt there would be a distinctly bad effect on her husband if anyone were to make a dramatic cross-country trip to his bedside (they live outside San Francisco, and he was in Boston's Peter Bent Brigham Hospital).

The only probable long-distance visitors were her mother-in-law, who lived with them and, while not an invalid, did need some attention—and their seventeen-year-old son, for whom she turned the negative "No, you cannot come," into a positive "Here's how you can help":

> He wanted to come—but I said, "No, I need you there. I'll need you there to help with Grandma. To keep her from worrying or trying to come, which would be too much for her."
> And we had animals to take care of, too.

Taking care of the family pets may seem ludicrously anticlimactic, but it is another thing *to be done* that the child can feel is a positive help. And, while taking care of Grandmother and keeping her from worrying about her own son may score more points on a child's I-am-helping meter than would walking Fido, the latter is better than "doing nothing" as a way to help. With a little ingenuity you can find *real* alternatives. Taking care of younger children, keeping them from disturbing their father, that sort of thing. If you are then appropriately lavish with your praise for how they are helping, even help-Daddy tasks that seem objectively inconsequential take on gratifying importance.

You will be pleased and proud of—yes, and touched by—the maturity, consideration, and affectionate concern your children display, the way they rise to the occasion. And it is easy to lose sight of the fact that they are children. If ninety-nine times they behave like adults—and refreshingly mature, sensible, and selfless adults, at that!—the next time they may still bring you up short by understandably being . . . children. It is no cause for dismay. It is just a reminder of what they are. And what you must allow them to remain. It is a mistake to push them too hard or too often into an adult role.

Nothing about raising children is simple, heart attack or no heart attack. But with your wits about you, and an appreciation of what the dangers are in the reaction of children to what is for them just another stress of growing up—it is not difficult.

In fact, if we have seemed to dwell on the subject of children's reactions to their father's heart attack, it is very likely because we are mothers. There really should not be much to worry about. Make sure they understand; make sure they are ready for a certain change in the way they eat, live, and make noise; make sure they know they are loved. Which, when you come down to it, applied long before the heart attack!

CHAPTER

14

Just What the Doctor Ordered

In Chapter Nine we gave you some advice that we expect you did not take: it is nearly impossible to keep from comparing notes with other Heart Wives on how long your respective husbands must stay in the hospital. Now we offer some more advice that forms a matched set with the other. It is unlikely that you will follow this, either, but who knows? You may be one Heart Wife who does manage to spare herself the unnecessary problems (and unhappiness) that comes of ignoring this advice. So here goes:

DO NOT COMPARE NOTES WITH ANY OTHER HEART WIFE ON ANY ASPECT OF YOUR HUSBAND'S TREATMENT.

Notice, we said "treatment." We are not talking about experiences, problems, emotions, and the like, but the prescriptions and proscriptions your husband receives from his doctor.

If the next Heart Wife you meet tells you all about the wonderful course of treatment her husband's doctor has prescribed and the astounding progress her husband is making, would you rush home to urge that treatment on your husband? Of course not. If it sounded so compellingly sensational you had to find out more about it, you would end up discussing it with your husband's doctor. And he would tell you one of three things: either the "wonder treatment" is too new and untested for him to want to risk using it on your husband, who is, after all, progressing very nicely (and what do you answer to that? "Oh, go on, chance it?"); or the treatment is not suited to your husband's case; or the treatment is perfectly sound and might very well suit your husband, but there is no reason to think it will afford any better or faster progress than he is already making.

So comparing treatments is literally useless; you cannot put the information you get to any practical use. Which means having it, knowing that some other treatment is helping some other man recover faster than your husband, can only be frustrating and disappointing. Do you really need any extra frustrations or disappointments in your life right now?

While a certain human element of faddism does exist in medical theories about the treatment of heart patients, there is always much more similarity than difference in the way one doctor will treat a patient and the way another doctor would treat the same patient. We had better emphasize that last part: the *same* patient. When Alice tells Zelda about the wonders her husband's cardiologist has performed, Zelda will fret over why her husband is not getting the same treatment. The answer is that Alice and Zelda are married to different men who have different conditions, different problems, and require different treatments.

If you start trading treatment and progress reports with Alice, Zelda, and other Heart Wives up and down the alphabet, certain things are bound to happen. You will find out that Alice's husband has a doctor who lets him do things you wish your husband could do: be more active, eat other things and sooner. Or you will find that Zelda's husband's doctor lets him do the same things your husband does, only a lot sooner: they had sex practically on the ride home from the hospital; her husband went back to work X amount of time after the attack, while your husband is still spending most of the day in bed. And if it should turn out that your husband is way ahead of Alice's and Zelda's husbands, you will no sooner start congratulating yourself (while making them feel rotten) than you will meet Betty and Yolande, whose husbands' recoveries will appear a headlong, pell-mell rush compared to what will suddenly and darkly seem the snail's crawl of your husband's progress.

That is when comparing notes can turn from useless to harmful, and you find yourself in the way of temptation. Why not, you tell yourself, find a doctor for your husband who can work the same sort of miracles. We tell you now, that doctor is hard to find. What's more, Alice and Zelda (or Betty and Yolande—or any of them, for that matter) have not been more clever at selecting doctors than you. If you want your husband to do what their husbands are doing, or to do it as soon as their husbands do it, what you need are their husbands, not their husbands' doctors. Your doctor would probably let Alice's husband do what his doctor lets him do, and let Zelda's husband do it as soon and as vigorously. And both of those doctors, if consulted, would have your husband on the same schedule (or near enough as to make no difference) as your own doctor does.

There are not only no miracles involved in the treatment of a heart patient (at least none you can count on or obtain through a cunning choice of doctors), there are also no particular mysteries or secrets. It is fashionable to say "Medicine is an art," which is largely true; what is untrue is to finish the catch phrase with . . . "not a science." Medicine is both art and science. That means it has some definite rules, definitive tests, and standard procedures. To use the old word, there are "specifics" for heart patients—medicines, treatments, and routines that have known and measurable results. The reason different doctors prescribe different treatments for different heart patients is because the patients are different. They have had heart attacks different in severity, in complications, in prognosis—in so many ways that the wonder is not that treatments differ but that they are similar. In fact, as your doctor will tell you, he prescribes different regimens for different patients of his own; and if he has a patient whose condition is like that of Alice's or Zelda's husbands, he is prescribing just about the same course of treatment, the same gradation of activity that their own doctors do.

Do just what the doctor orders. In both senses of "just" —exactly and only. Encourage your husband to do the same. Your doctor may not always "know best," but he assuredly knows *better* than you do. And better than your husband does. And better than Alice, Zelda, all the Heart Wives in between, plus—surprise!—their doctors. That's right. If your husband's doctor happens to be a first-year resident in cardiology, he knows more about the proper treatment for your husband than every other doctor in the world *who has not examined your husband*. The catch, of course, is in italics. Put that way, it is obvious. Unfortunately, the virtues of another doctor are seldom put that way to us. It is always in terms of the wonders he has done for his patients. We all want so desperately to have our husbands achieve the fastest, most complete recovery, any inkling we get of a doctor who works—there is no other word—*miracles* can make us feel we are inflicting second-rate care on our husbands if we do not rush to consult The Doctor.

All this may sound as though we are starry-eyed handmaidens to the American Medical Association. Do we urge worshipful acceptance of whatever doctor you happen to start with? Not even close to it. We have done some doctor-switching, ourselves. There are times and occasions when it is only good sense to want another doctor for your husband. None of the reasons, however, have anything to do with not accepting what the doctor tells you is a proper and safe course of treatment. Far from it! The best and most common reason for wanting another doctor is if the one you have seems to take a cavalier attitude toward your husband's recovery or toward any possible signs of a recurrence. If some night your husband has chest pains and (typically, over his objections) you call his doctor only to hear some variation on the exasperating theme of "Take two aspirin and call me in the morning" (the most common is "Oh, it's probably gas or maybe a slight kidney reaction; I'll check him at my office—*tomorrow*"), start looking for another doctor. And do not wait for morning. Even if it turns out that, yes, this time it was just a little gas or whatever, you still want another doctor. One who does not diagnose by mental telepathy or practice long-distance medicine. You want a doctor who would rather answer false alarms than ever be late for a single fire. Of course, if you demand that sort of reaction—which you should—you have a responsibility not to consciously be "crying wolf" all the time. But any cardiologist who objects to being called out of bed at night should give serious thought to switching specialties.

Another excellent reason to switch doctors is if your husband expresses any lack of confidence in the doctor you have. We include this because, as they say, anything is possible. Actually, though, the opposite is much more often the case: you will have a lack of confidence and your husband will be happy as a clam with the doctor he has. A man who has been through a heart attack and is now on the way to recovery will tend to credit everyone within a ten-mile radius of the hospital with having saved his life. Heart Wives have told us of instances in which a doctor sounded suspiciously like an incompetent. But their husbands (who recovered in spite of the doctor—or, more probably, because of the marvels available in a CCU, the routine competence of most CCU staffs, and the heart's astounding resiliency and toughness) still wanted to stick with "the doctor they had come through with." It is enough to choke you with emotion. Or something.

For instance, a couple we'll call Mr. and Mrs. N had moved to another state only sixteen months before the attack and had no regular doctor. So when Mr. N had a heart attack, his wife called a friend from the hospital to ask for the name of a cardiologist. She got four warm recommendations and simply called the first on the list. As luck would have it, the doctor was on vacation, but his young associate was ready to leap right in and take over. Mr. N may have been the first cardiac case the associate had ever handled all on his own. That was Mrs. N's impression, anyway:

> He was like an iceberg. Except once he came out and acted real scared, as though we were going to lose my husband. And he said, "I don't know, I don't know! I can't control . . ." What's the word? fibrillation? "I can't control it, I can't control it—it won't stabilize!" And he looked it.
>
> I finally said [*very small voice*], "Is he going to be all right?"
>
> When you come out and *say* it, you're pretty scared! And you know what he said? "I don't know."

By that time, a friend of Mrs. N's had gotten to the hospital. On hearing this less than inspiring exchange, she said, "Why don't you call the next name on the list?" Mrs. N did and the other doctor was wonderful. *But.* It was about three weeks before her husband could be convinced to let the younger doctor find someone else to practice on—and only after Mrs. N agreed to write a letter both to the doctor and his senior partner praising him as a brilliant medical man, a sterling humanitarian, and a benefactor to all who ail, plus alleging some "family connection" with the other doctor (whom, of course, they had not known existed beforehand).

Your personal feelings about the doctor do not enter into it. Had the young associate been three times the "iceberg" (which is actually one of the prettier names Mrs. N had for him), she would not have cared, so long as he was competent. If your husband is "in good hands," it does not really matter that you might not want to shake one of them.

That was the case with another Heart Wife, who told us:

> I had a really bad relationship with this doctor. He had been my doctor, and I had left him because I didn't like him.
>
> But my husband had stayed with him. They went to college together, and they were "old buddies."
>
> Well, he really had my husband's best interest in mind and he brought in all the best specialists and everything.
>
> I just don't . . . *relate* well with him.

But my husband likes him and has confidence in him, and
that's what counts. It isn't that he's a bad doctor; I guess he's fine.
It's his personality I can't stand.

You do not have to "stand" the doctor. All that counts is the
doctor's competence, and your husband's confidence in him.

The reverse is also true. A doctor can be Mr. Personality
himself—you and your husband may count him among your
closest friends; but if he clearly cannot do the job, you must get
another doctor, no matter how much you hate hurting him.

The only other legitimate reason for switching doctors is the
kind of doctor you had at the time of the attack. If he is a general
practitioner, it is probably unnecessary to switch; he will want
to call in a cardiologist himself. (If he does not, you should—and
quickly. Then start looking for a GP with better judgment,
which will not be hard to find.) The sticky point comes when
your regular doctor is an internist who "does a little heart work
on the side." Then it depends on how much actual cardiology
experience he has. Many "internists" are really cardiac
specialists who also practice internal medicine, mostly as an
accommodation for their patients. Perhaps even more important, it depends on how much confidence you have always had
in him as a doctor and as a human being of good judgment and
professional pride. If you completely trust his judgment, leave it
up to him; he will have too much professionalism in him to let his
own vanity keep your husband from getting the best possible
treatment. He will know what he can handle and what he
cannot—and will call for a specialist in anything like a close
decision.

Of course, if you are in any doubt, you can always say the
magic words: "I'd like to have a specialist in for consultation."
No doctor can object to that, especially if you put it in terms of
"You know what trust we have in you as our doctor, but I just
won't feel that I've done everything I should unless I know that
someone who's a specialist has checked him; you understand
don't you?" He will understand. You are frightened and want
reassurance. It is no insult to him, nor will he take it as one.

Naturally, there is a limit to calling in specialists. Doctor-shopping is ridiculous. If the course of your husband's recovery is smooth and reasonably swift and you have confidence in your doctor—and especially if your husband feels the same way—it is folly to ask for consultations. (Highly expensive folly, by the way!) Your doctor will (rightly) resent it, or at least be mightily puzzled. And so will the specialist! In Chapter Twenty we discuss situations in which you must forget everything but your husband and your family; but unless you have a taste for gothic relationships, there is no reason to go about offending people on whom, after all, you are depending. Doctors *are* human, just like everyone; and although we sincerely believe professional pride would make a doctor who felt insulted still do his level best, do you really *want* your husband's well-being and speedy recovery (maybe, life) in disgruntled hands?

If you start doctor-shopping or doctor-switching every time the doctor says your husband should wait another week before getting up or going for walks or returning to work, you may find it a little difficult to locate competent doctors who are willing even to talk to you.

To sum up: there is nothing wrong in switching doctors if you are convinced that the one you have simply cannot handle the case. In any event, there is nothing wrong with asking for a consulting specialist to look at your husband.

On the other hand, there is nothing right about chivvying the doctor to treat your husband the way Alice's or Zelda's doctors treat their husbands; take action because you are worried, not because you are envious.

Do not ask for a different treatment.

Do not substitute your own notions for the doctor's on the subject of diet and activity (any more than you would substitute your own ideas for his about medication).

Still less should you substitute another doctor's ideas that have come to you, through however glowing a description of her husband's progress, from another Heart Wife.

In short, do just what your doctor *ordered.*

A Little Egg Yolk Won't Kill Him;
A Lot of Fussing Might

Do what your doctor orders, but don't be Prussian about it. Following the doctor's orders yet not being fanatical or getting hysterical when minor lapses occur are instructions that should be inseparably fixed in your mind, constantly modifying each other.

Certainly, your husband should cut out food and activities his doctor specifies and cut down on those his doctor says to limit. What's more, he should stick to whatever limits the doctor sets.

Certainly, you should help your husband follow the doctor's orders.

But just as certainly, the atmosphere in which he follows the orders is nearly as important as the orders themselves, and a good deal more important than absolute observance of each little order.

Nothing can sour the atmosphere faster than a wife who becomes a sort of warden, strictly metering each moment of exercise, gimlet-eyed at mealtimes to make sure her husband does not have one calorie, one milligram of saturated fat over the daily allowance. Few men marry women because of their un-canny resemblance to an Army sergeant. That sort of hawklike wariness does not even help. In the long run it often produces exactly the results a wife is trying to guard against.

As one Heart Wife said:

> If you are going to hound him, you're going to add pressures by destroying your relationship. Ultimately, you're going to have to leave it up to him anyway.
>
> Every time I think he's eating too much, I don't necessarily say something. Or if he asks for a dessert, or something with lots of calories?—I give it to him. Usually it's in the house, because the kids eat things.
>
> If he says, "Don't we have any ice cream?"—well, yes, we have ice cream. I know it's a futile battle pretending there isn't.

Because if he wants it bad enough, he'll get in the car and go get it!

And he does want it bad enough, sometimes. He knows better. But I can't make it *my* battle constantly. It's his battle.

All you can ever reasonably hope to do is help him win the battle. If you try to fight it for him, you will end up fighting, not the battle, but him. And, besides creating damaging tensions, you can drive him to deliberately overstepping the line of common sense, simply as a matter of defiance. "Just for the sake of argument we'll see who's going to tell who what to do and and what not to do." You know how it goes—and how easily it can start.

We suspect some lingering sense of denial is involved, especially in the years to come. In mid-swallow of something he is perfectly aware is a coronary folly, he may be relishing the *idea* of ice cream as much as the tutti-frutti itself. For a moment he is indulging himself by doing something he would be able to do without a second thought—but for the heart attack.

Just as there may be that lingering trace of denial, so his now forgotten hostility toward you can revive if, every second, you give him the feeling that you are watching and waiting, ready to pounce at the first sign of wavering from the straight line of the doctor's instructions.

From your point of view, the problem is a natural tendency to overreact to dangers your husband may face (even when he himself is creating the dangers). If you get all tense and bothered at the notion that a speck of cholesterol may pass his lips, you tend to do things and say things that will make him pretty tense, too. But not with anything like the result you want. He will become tense about you, not the broken rule.

During a conversation with one Heart Wife we found ourselves edging nervously to a position perilously close to that wrong and wrongheaded panic over what amounts to a trifle compared to the tensions that can come of treating trifles with high seriousness. We had been discussing polyunsaturates with Mrs. F, who is quite expert in the field of, as she called it, "coronary cuisine." In listening to the tape we made of that chat, we are ashamed at the note of genuine alarm we hear on our part. We must have been about ready to rush home and destroy every vestige of corn oil we could find:

Mrs. F: Well, actually, corn oil is more saturated than your safflower oil. Your saf. and your soy are least saturated and with the highest balance of polyunsaturates.
H.W.C.: [*worried*] Really?!! You mean corn oil isn't okay to—
Mrs. F: It's not important. We're talking about very small differences here. I just happen to know there is a difference at all because I looked up the saturation on the different oils.
H.W.C.: You're sure it's all right to use the corn—
Mrs. F: Oh, yes! The amount of difference is minimal—and you don't use enough of any for there to be a dangerous difference. . . .

A little later on we remarked on what a blow it had been for us to hear that shellfish had been discovered to be positively teeming with cholesterol, because it had been such a favorite. We asked Mrs. F what she had done about it:

Mrs. F: I think the sensible thing is to serve them, but not often. Once in a while I'll have shrimp—just not as any kind of a regular thing. Actually, if you're moderate, it doesn't really matter. I haven't checked if there are any recent developments or conflicts; I generally call up the Heart Association every once in a while and say, "What's new?"
Mainly, you just use common sense about it and be moderate. If we go out and my husband orders lobster, well, fine—I don't even open my mouth, anymore. I used to—but I don't anymore. So, instead of making a fuss, I cut down somewhere else that week. Two eggs instead of three. It's just common sense.

That's what it is, all right! Moderation and common sense. To keep after your husband, bugging him about each morsel he eats, each ounce of weight he picks up (in his hands or around his middle), each drop of sweat on his forehead when he exercises, each minute he works late or stays up late—those things keep him off-balance and on edge. Reminding him in a restaurant or at a party, embarrassing him, has to be harder on him and his heart than the occasional lobster he might eat or the "one too many" he might drink. It is endless fussing about an extra egg that can do the real damage—much more of it and much more quickly than the egg yolk itself.

Be moderate. Use common sense. Keep a sense of perspective and of values. It means the watchword is moderation in *all* things—including how immoderately you try to keep him moderate.

CHAPTER

15

This Is Your Lives

We would like to tell you a joke.

There were two sparrows sitting on a fence. Being especially dim sparrows, they did not move from that fence. Ever. The summer sun beat down on them; they choked in the dust, panted with thirst, ached with sunburn. And still they sat there. In winter they shivered with cold, shook with chills, their feathers drooping and soggy in the snow and rain.

This went on for years.

Finally one sparrow turned to the other and croaked hoarsely "This sure is a rotten way to live, isn't it?"

The second sparrow's brow furrowed in thought. Then he turned to his companion and asked, "Compared to what?"

From the moment your husband had his heart attack he has had a "cardiac condition." He stopped being a heart patient when he left the hospital; he stops recovering from a heart attack when he is back doing, full time, whatever he did before the heart attack. But he will never stop being a man with a cardiac condition. And for the rest of your life together, you will be the wife of a man with a cardiac condition.

A rotten way to live?

Compared to what? Certainly not compared to the alterna-

tive—pretending he has no heart condition. If either of you did
that, it would not end the condition; but it is an outstanding way
to end his life.

Compared to the way you were living? Well, something
about it—or a combination of somethings—gave your husband a
heart attack and has been giving you a fair number of problems
ever since. That's good? The only reasonable conclusion is,
whatever way you were living before, the way you live from
now on cannot have a worse result. Besides, you have not tried
it yet. At least you have had only the bad; the good part is about
to begin. So let's look at the sort of life, or the variety of lives,
you can expect to live as a cardiac couple.

Your husband's despondency and a large measure of his
hostility when he was in the hospital and when he first got home
was the result of his assumptions about life as a permanent
"cardiac case." It seemed a rotten way to live. And this much is
true: it is permanent.

So firmly and affirmatively realize that whatever the quality
of the life you live as a cardiac couple, it is not a sometime thing.
It *is* permanent. And it is a different sort of life from whatever
you have had.

The question is, different *how?* Start with the difference in
your life. You are a Heart Wife.

A woman we know developed a severe case of diabetes in her
late thirties. She had always been highly active, had five children
and a large house to run; she also had most of a master's degree
in city planning—acquired *after* the diabetes, when she found
herself getting a little bored. We asked her whether diabetes
had made much of a difference in how she lives. After ponder-
ing, she said, "Well . . . yes; now I take insulin."

Exactly. She takes insulin. And she does not take certain
other things: cake, candy, anything with a discernible sugar
content. That may suggest that she does not take dessert; it
depends on whether or not she has taken the time to plan ahead
and the trouble to make an allowed dessert for herself. If she is
going on a trip, or planning to be away from home all day, she

must make some plan to be sure she has a supply of food with her
and a supply of insulin and syringes.

It is no big deal—if she plans.

Now you take thought about certain things. You plan. You
learn. Sometimes you scheme. As one Heart Wife put it, "I
learned to be a little crafty."

What she was being crafty about illuminates the sort of
planning a Heart Wife must be prepared to do. It makes a world
of difference in how comfortable your new life-style will be.

She and her husband were out of town at the time of his
attack. They had left the wet, cold, and windy Chicago winter
for a sales-convention-cum-vacation in warm, sunny San
Diego. After the attack they decided to stay on until spring.

Their children were grown; their responsibilities were relatively few. In fact, the only negative was that their friends and
relatives couldn't see him. But for her, that was a compelling
plus; her husband is the kind of man who automatically reacts to
any social stimulus, who cannot sit back and watch.

They had moved from the hospital to a cheery efficiency
apartment on the bay ("If I'm honest," she said, "I have to tell
you, I could have gone on like that for the rest of my life!"). And
they had a fine time as he recuperated, with nothing to do but
rest and enjoy each other. Then it was April and time to go
home:

> The day before, I put some things in a bag, and we went to a
> small hotel; if Harry was in the apartment when I was getting
> everything ready for the move—or even if I had someone in to do
> the work—he'd feel he had to pitch in and pack and lift. Or else
> I'd have to bitch at him about not straining, and he'd feel bad. Or
> he'd just sit and watch, and feel worse—because there's, you
> know, the right way, wrong way, and Harry's way to do
> anything; he hates feeling . . . "left out."
>
> So there we were in the hotel, and the landlady at the apart-
> ment and her son took care of everything.
>
> But what I really had to worry about was, okay—he's got a
> good start; now we get back, and we won't have a foot in the

door before it's going to start: the visits. The relatives, the good
buddies. They've missed him and they have to show him they
miss him. That would ruin the good start we had toward his
recovery.

So, maybe a week, ten days before, I wrote that we are
coming home on such-and-such a date. And we'll let everyone
know the flight in plenty of time to get the brass band together.

Then we flew in three days ahead—and I didn't even want to
tell the airline our right names!

Once back home, she let a few people at a time know they
were back and so managed to space out the expected flood of
visitors.

That kind of planning *is* hard because it involves such a
wide-ranging combination of insights and abilities. It means
studying your husband until you can predict with nearly a
clairvoyant's accuracy just what his reactions will be in different
circumstances. Maybe you can do that now. But it is only the
start. You must also be able to recognize situations that require
planning-for, and spot them enough ahead of time to make your
planning effective. Then you must have (or develop) a talent for
whatever manipulative and strategic action is necessary to
implement the plans you concoct.

In the early stages, the first months after he comes home,
your objective is to eliminate any experiences or situations you
know will create tension or extreme anger or stress for your
husband. That is a matter of physical necessity. But it is even
more necessary for him to confront those same situations later in
his recovery. Anywhere from six months to a year after the
attack, your emphasis should start to shift from trying to
eliminate tensions to simply trying to avoid the more exacer-
bating ones.

Two years after the attack, at the outside, you should not
have to take any extraordinary measures to shield your husband
from the normal knocks of living. By then, you and he will have
firmly established for yourselves a sensible "cardiac couple"

life-style that gives you maximum satisfaction—with minimum risks.

Let's look at the elements that bring you and your husband to this point, and some of the problems that can get in the way.

Once your husband is up and about—even when he is apparently back on a normal schedule—there will still be many things both of you know he should not do. Some will be just a matter of common sense, others will be a matter of doctor's orders.

Most, of both kinds, will result in what we call "Suitcase Problems." They get their name from one of the first instances of the problem for many Heart Wives. One of them described it like this:

> When my husband was in the hospital, I used to think about how will he feel and how will I feel when we're, say, going on a vacation, and I'm picking up the suitcases?
>
> Now, anyone—myself included—has to think that's the silliest thing I ever heard. Worrying about something like *that!* Except . . . you say it to someone else with a husband who had a heart attack, and they say . . . "You, too!"

They are not physical problems. So no physical solution for them is possible. In fact, more often than not, there is no solution at all.

Consider how another Heart Wife tried to devise one:

> I always made sure any suitcases were packed and ready to go enough ahead of time so I could get them out—in someone else's hands—before he was ready to go. The kids, at home; a bell-boy—anyone!

The trouble is, however crafty a solution that seems to be, it is a solution to the wrong problem! The problem is not getting suitcases from here to there, it is who does the "getting." The point of this whole class of "Suitcase Problems" is the unhappy and demoralizing effect of your taking over a masculine role (however necessarily, however reluctantly) at the very time when so many elements in your husband's life conspire to build a crisis of masculinity for him. The remarks of the doctor/patient we quoted before are so to the point, we would remind you of them again: You have to understand that this is a terribly emasculating experience. He is just there, lying there helpless, and he wonders, am I still even a man?

Another aspect of these problems is the spottiness with which they appear. Some men set no great store by suitcase-lifting as a sign of masculinity, but are mortified by being driven places by their wives.

There is no way of telling, beforehand, how big a worry loss of masculinity will be, or how long it will be one. It has no relation to objective fact, nor has it any relation to how concerned or unconcerned he was about it before his heart attack. Some men are more worried than others, that's all. But then, so are some wives. You and your husband may not even be worried about the same things. While you fret over his (and your) reaction to picking up suitcases, he may be disturbed only by your taking over som household function, like making out checks for monthly bills. Or he may find everything you worry about a challenge to his masculinity—plus some things you had not worried about and would not dream could represent to him any potential loss of masculinity.

For instance, one Heart Wife who was delighted that her husband didn't mind being driven, later told us that one of her biggest problems, in the early stages of recovery was his constant "forgetting" to take nitroglycerin along with him when he went out. The doctor had prescribed it in case of possible, lingering angina pains.

> When he first came home from the hospital, he didn't want to carry the nitroglycerin with him. He didn't want to admit he might have to take it.
> I knew he'd never carry it around. And I knew he related it to seeing his mother always popping it. That looked like an invalid, and he wasn't going to be that.

That was part of it, surely, but only part. It seems pretty clear that he felt that being required to carry a "pill box," being dependent on a supply of medicine, was emasculating. He was not going to do it, even at the risk of suffering otherwise totally unnecessary pain, or worse. If there is any doubt that this was a crisis of masculinity, consider his wife's solution:

> Actually, he only needed it just once. We were out walking, and there was a flutter. And that's when it came to a head.
>
> I said, "Let's stop—now's the time you take it."
>
> And he said, "I don't need it." And we walked on a little further, and he said, "Oooo—I feel a little dizzy."
>
> I'd been carrying the tube in my purse, so I got it out and he took it.
>
> We talked about it later—and it was really out in the open. I said, "I really understand how you feel about it. But will I have to tag along everywhere you go, carrying it in my purse the rest of my days? Because that's the only way I'll be comfortable if you won't take it with you."
>
> Well, he carries it all the time now. He never needs it, but he carries it, because he knows it makes me comfortable that I know if he ever needs it, he'll have it.

Once he was doing it for her, to calm *her* fears, carrying pills lost much of its emasculating significance. Enough, anyway, so that he could do it comfortably.

At first, "Do it for me" may seem a cure-all technique for the entire spectrum of "Suitcase Problems."

Unfortunately, as with most cure-alls, you are lucky if it cures any, let alone all, problems. It certainly will not work for any problem where switching masculine and feminine roles involves activities that cut deep to the core of a man's self-image. If he must change jobs, for instance, with you becoming the main source of family income, even for a short while, a "Do it for me" won't assuage his gloom.

There is no cure-all for "Suitcase Problems," neither the trivial ones nor the serious ones. But there is a way to think about them that may help.

You are a woman and you can and will do whatever is necessary to keep your man alive and well. They need not make you any less feminine. They are temporary measures. You never treat them as permanent; you never usurp willingly or eagerly any of his roles as man, husband, or father. You let him know you need him, you rely on him, you cannot *wait* (but you *will* wait, patiently) for him to feel again totally himself. That is *feel*—not *be*. Because, in every sense that counts, he has not been any less the man you married.

The emphatic note, here, is on the word *temporary*. That is the word you must immediately attach to even the thought of role-changing. And *permanent* must be the word both you and your husband should have in mind when thinking about his cardiac condition. The need for this combination of attitudes suggests still another drawback to "Do it for me" as an effective, long-range technique (even if it would work). There are too many dangerous implications in it for his ultimate adjustment and for your future lives. He cannot get in the habit of doing things he should be doing "for you." Because what he should be doing in the way of diet, exercise, resting, and the like are the necessary context of a successful adjustment to living well and long with a cardiac condition.

Once you fall into the trap of finding an external reason for every action or self-denial (take your pills, dear, because I will worry if you don't; give up smoking, because the children object to tobacco; let's go for your daily walk, because I feel like going for a walk now), there is no way out. If you must endlessly find reasons for your husband to do what is necessary, you will be all but living his life for him. And no one has enough time to live two full lives. Your husband must live his own life, and he must come to a state of mind in which he willingly, of his own accord, does what is necessary to go on living it.

Naturally, we are talking about a long-term attitude. In the first months after his heart attack the important thing is what he does, not why he does it. Anything goes. But, conning, jollying, wheedling—and, yes, nagging—are only expedients. You must recognize them as such, and realize how unsatisfactory they are for any sort of sensible, years-on-end life. Like role-switching, they must be seen as highly temporary.

We know a Heart Wife who is ready to do everything she can for her husband. She is almost fiercely selfless. Yet she stated the long-term problem with ultimate force and clarity:

> He's one of those guys who doesn't always do what he's supposed to.
>
> He should be walking, he should be resting, he should be doing all kinds of things. He doesn't do these things unless I do them.
>
> Maybe that's par for the course.
>
> But they've got to learn that we can't take care of them all their lives.
>
> Maybe we don't feel like walking every five minutes. But, say, in the evening, if you're going out, it takes us an hour to get dressed—and maybe it takes them five minutes.
>
> Well, he could be walking while I'm getting dressed. It's one of those things—and there are lots of them.

There are really two related problems here. Many men will depend on their wives for a push to do what heart patients must do. It is not the same as becoming a cardiac cripple, it is almost a reversion to denial, a most insidious form of denial, since it feeds the masculine ego. He will get his rest and take his exercise and watch his weight—for you, not because he has to. It is somehow manly not to take care of himself, or at least unmanly to seem concerned enough with his health to take care of it. (If you doubt that, check on the trend of men's overshoe sales at the nearest department store.) But he will readily fall in with any suggestion from his wife that he is following the doctor's orders to please her, and not because he perceives any necessity about the orders. He will "humor the little woman."

You can see how important it is that "Do it for me" should as quickly as possible become "Do it because you know it will help you live; do it for *yourself,* as well as for me, the children, and everyone else who loves you." Those, finally, are the only terms on which your husband can make a permanent accommodation to life with a cardiac condition.

That is what you are striving for, the life of an avowed "cardiac couple." Your husband should be able to say, unflinchingly, "I have a heart condition." You should be able to say, "I am a Heart Wife." It is not a litany that must be repeated every morning; maybe you will not ever actually say the words. No matter—as long as you both act them out.

The need for automatic observance of the ground rules of life as a cardiac couple is the reason for the attitude expressed in Chapter Fourteen. It cannot depend on "who's watching." Because no one will be watching all the time, or even a meaningful portion of the time. So if you turn it into some sort of a contest, pouncing on him at every infraction, the logical next step is for him to think of all heart-condition rules as being something to observe only when someone is there to blow the whistle.

Up to now we have been talking about problems. How about pleasures?

If you are like most Heart Wives we know, you will find that the pleasures of your life as a cardiac couple are not merely now-and-then compensations for the problems, but the dominant factor. The "statistics" we are about to give are totally unreliable from any mathematical viewpoint. But we are convinced the spirit behind them is an accurate reflection of reality.

Over 90 percent of the Heart Wives we have talked to whose husbands had heart attacks two or more years ago feel that their lives are better now, their marriages stronger now, and that they and their husbands are better adjusted and happier now than before the attack.

Less than 5 percent felt their lives, marriages, etc., were not satisfactory. And of those, most felt their "etc." were no great shakes before the heart attack, either.

The remainder felt that while the aftermath of the heart attack had not made anything noticeably better for them, their husbands were somewhat better off.

One Heart Wife told us:

> We found out, for the first time in our lives—as individuals, and together in our married life—we found out what was important and what wasn't important. Before, we took everything for granted. Each other, too. And the children. All at once, you can't take anything for granted. So you stop and think.
> We do much better now. Every way!

Does that strike you as a trifle too hip-hip-hooray? Especially since we are talking about the results of today's most serious medical problem? We do not blame you. We have felt that way, too, and we have said as much. For instance:

MRS. A: The year after his heart attack, we went to Europe. He finally decided he's going to do the whole thing, everything he always talked about. Now! At last! You know—"I'm going to do what I want to *do*—and to hell with making a little more money just so I can pay bigger taxes!"

I'm sure every woman tells you the same thing—that it changed her husband's attitude about everything. His whole approach to life.

And I think it's so much healthier! If they only had that attitude before, maybe they wouldn't get the heart attacks in the first place. You only live once. You can only make so much money, anyway—and why, if you don't have time to enjoy it? Why should it take a heart attack to make a man see that?

H.W.C.: I don't know. But I wouldn't want anybody to have a heart attack just to find out how to live.

MRS. A: Well, I would! If *that's* what it takes—because the other isn't living.

I've seen it in so many men with heart attacks! They don't *start* to live until they nearly die.

I don't mean just the trip, for my husband. Everything! How he lives and enjoys it now—he even enjoys his work more now.

She was right. There is no denying that in many ways you and your husband are leading more sensible, richer lives as a result of the adjustments you make to life as a cardiac couple. Start with the physical aspects of your lives.

We have already discussed nutrition. And there cannot be two different minds on the subject; with reasonable ease you will be eating more healthfully, and feeling better because of it, than ever before.

Your husband must lead a more physically active life—and you can join him if you like. It is true that we do not always feel like going for a walk every five minutes, not even every day perhaps. But his physical need to go for walks can be a boon to your marriage.

We are told that "The family that prays together stays together." Maybe, but it depends on how long they stick around to talk with one another before and after. On the other hand, we can guarantee the validity of this: "The couple that walks together, talks together." And walking will be, certainly at the start, a principal form of exercise, then amusement. It is a great time to talk. (At least on the flat and downslopes; when you both get used to it, maybe even uphill.) After a while consider biking, which is getting very chic, nowadays, so you won't even feel at all odd. And you do get to see more.

One word of caution, though. From a Heart Wife:

> We were lucky. From the time he came home, everything was just—you know, up, up, up! All except one little scare.
>
> It wasn't really a pain, just kind of a . . . feeling. But what made me mad was, it wasn't necessary at all.
>
> The thing was, nobody told us—they said, okay, you should do regular walking. But they didn't tell us you're supposed to wait an hour after dinner, like with swimming. And this one night, we went right after a big dinner—to walk it off, you know—and wham!

That one caution, aside, you will find walking together a most enjoyable form of exercise. You may be having so much fun, so openly, even the children will want to join in.

And speaking of children . . .

Despite the problems we have already discussed in previous chapters, most Heart Wives feel that the problem-sharing spirit of solidarity that any crisis like a heart attack creates has brought their children closer to them and their husbands. As you might expect it to do.

But what if you have no children now? Or if you had been planning to have more children? There are many reasons to go right ahead with your plans. First of all there is your husband's morale. Having a child will probably help it immeasurably, as one Heart Wife told us she discovered to her intense surprise:

> We weren't planning it, but I became pregnant a year after the attack. And I was scared to death when I learned that I was pregnant.
>
> It was something that we had wanted before. But . . . now? Anyway, he was very happy about it.
>
> In fact, my husband felt really terrific during this time. I carried through to my seventh month—but I didn't make it all the way through that time.
>
> I had worried a great deal about how he would go through delivery and whatever. And, of course, when I was rushed to the hospital and it was actually a still-birth, then I wondered how he was going to take it—even though I was very depressed myself.
>
> He went through that entire time very well. He didn't seem to have pangs or anything.

Of course he was delighted at the news of the pregnancy! What better antidote for any crisis of masculinity could there be? And even the sad termination of the pregnancy had a beneficial side that is not altogether surprising: helping his wife through the difficult shock was surely a bracing change from self-worries and self-doubts. And just from the typical self-absorption of cardiac patients.

We do not mean to suggest that it is open-and-shut, that there is simply no question about whether you should have children, or more children, after the heart attack. At a post-hospital meeting of heart patients alone (that is, without their wives present), a young man in his mid twenties said that at the time of his attack he and his wife had just about decided they were well-enough launched in the world, financially, to start a family. The attack changed that. At least it did for her. He still wanted children, but she did not. He said they had discussed it and that she was perfectly honest about her reasons. Quoting our notes of the meeting:

> She was very much afraid to have children. She was afraid he would have another heart attack and she would end up raising the children alone.
>
> Also, was it right to raise children when their father would have to restrict his activities and perhaps not be the sort of father he wants to be?

An older man at the meeting said something that bears strongly on the point: "We made up our minds we were going to live, and enjoy life."

Another Heart Wife told us approximately the same thing:

> The hardest decision was determining whether or not we should have another child. I always felt I didn't want to take on any huge commitments that will create a lot of pressure for him.
>
> But we decided—Yes. We did not want to give up that delight.
>
> And I'm glad we did.

Frankly, we are a little ill at ease, maybe somewhat embarrassed, discussing this problem. In a way, we were so lucky, we should be disqualified from having an opinion. We both had as many children as we had planned to when our husbands had their heart attacks. The children were old enough, and our husbands made rapid enough recoveries, so there was very little question of them not participating in the children's lives. It's easy enough for *us* to talk. But we do feel that "not giving up that delight" says it all. And not only about children. One Heart Wife gave what seems to us a general answer to this and similar specific questions:

I was in mortal fear of losing my husband.

I had a very idealistic attitude toward my marriage, a very old-fashioned one in the light of the way the world goes now. And I could not tolerate the idea of my being alive without him.

And therefore . . . I could not permit myself the time to think, or the emotion to think, that he would die, or could die, and that I would be faced with living alone, without him.

And so I decided I was not going to waste any energy or time on that. I was going to make our lives as interesting and as pleasurable and as exciting—under the circumstances in which we were—as I could. And that was my goal.

And I think, in some ways, I was able to achieve it.

Doesn't that seem pretty sensible as the ultimate goal for any Heart Wife? It means, among other things, helping bring your husband around to a point of view that embraces a sane, satisfying view of himself, his work, his family, and the place that all have in relation to one another.

Generally speaking, there *is* a "cardiac personality." There are exceptions, of course, but men with coronaries quite often are among the more driving, tense, and compulsive people. The experience of a heart attack goes a long way toward helping such a man change. At a group meeting of cardiac couples, one man said:

Mr. U: No one has assurance you're going to live on and on. You just live your life as best you can.

H.W.C.: Do you think the heart attack has taken the fun out of it, out of life?

Mr. U: Well, I don't know. I do think you take life a little more seriously. You think about it a little more.

Mr. C: I think it changes people's outlook. And this is where, eventually, you have people coming to settle down and realize what things really are.

I mean they get a grip on themselves and start saying, "Well, this is reality; this is the way things really are. And *this* is important—living happy." Whereas all those

material things and power and being a big shot don't do
it for you anymore.

You grow up a lot—without gray hairs.

So the answer to maturity is . . . go have a heart
attack! [*laughter*]

Well, you and your husband don't have much choice: he had
the heart attack. Now you can capitalize on his maturing attitude by consciously playing the role of moderating influence.
Remember that the Heart Wife who was glad they decided to
have another child hesitated only because she did not want to
"create pressures for her husband." She went on to say:

> I'm still reluctant to take any steps that will be a major
> economic commitment, month by month.
>
> I have been steadfast in saying we're not adding rooms to the
> house and we're not buying a bigger house.
>
> There's some pressure to do this. Two of the boys share a
> room, and it would be nice if they each had a room. But it's that
> kind of long-range commitment that might turn out to be a drain
> that I'm wary of.
>
> My husband is very expansive, a very outgoing person, and he
> would say, "Oh, what the heck—we'll do it!" I'm much more
> conservative.
>
> I don't feel I'm sacrificing anything. And I feel my life is
> pretty much what I want it. I just don't want to create any
> enormous pressures that don't have to be created.
>
> I feel in his case it's the emotional thing that's dangerous; and
> a big financial commitment would be dangerous for him.
>
> What happens is—well, we've just been through landscaping.
> Now he decided we needed a new desk in our bedroom. And he
> kept saying, "Call up so-and-so and have him come out and give
> us a bid."
>
> Well, I know that a bid means the job is going to be done.
>
> So—I just haven't called up! That's all. I figure—let's get
> finished with the landscaping, and pay for it. Then we'll worry
> about the desk. That's my approach. I just stall a little bit.
>
> And he's busy, and not really thinking about it. But if we talk,
> he realizes I'm right.

Even men who drove themselves to coronaries can *learn* to take satisfaction from things short of empires—like having and enjoying children, having a pleasant time just living. But your part as moderating influence is essential in the learning process—even if there seems to be little chance of it making much impression on your husband. And even if your husband *must* build empires, it's important that you let him know you do not need them—you need him. It may not work. But he needs to know how you feel, so there is less pressure on him.

It all goes back to a basic shift in life orientation. When the sum of your different lives adds up to that of a cardiac couple, you will have learned, both of you, to "take it easy." One Heart Wife told us she felt one of the greatest lessons she and her husband had learned from the attack was just that: a nonpanic approach to living, even when it involved meeting crises. And it is a deeply satisfying moment when a Heart Wife realizes that, yes, now her husband is able to take in stride things that before would have, well, given him a heart attack! One Heart Wife whose husband is an accountant gave this example:

> Last week the phone rang at, oh, some ungodly hour—three, four—and it was a client. Hysterical. "It's awful, horrible, the end of the world!" He just got a call from the fire department—his place had burned down and all the records were probably up in smoke, and now what's gonna happen?
>
> Okay, three years ago it would have been like five minutes and Charlie would have been out of the house, driving like a crazy man to get there.
>
> Now, I was so proud of him! He said, "Okay, we'll go over everything in the morning. There's nothing to do now anyway." And—back to sleep! I knew he was more relaxed. But I didn't dream he was this far along. It's great!

Another Heart Wife told us in admiration how her husband had taken his father's death. On the way to the funeral he said:

> I'm going to stay as loose and cool as I can—and you remind me. Because, when Mother died, you know what happened, the way I took it.

She certainly did know. Two years before, her husband had had a second, though minor, heart attack—after more than five years of splendid recovery, and it happened a few weeks following his mother's funeral. He had learned. The hard way, maybe, but any way counts. And this time there was no heart attack.

You will change as well. It will happen sooner or later. And you will find, like most Heart Wives, that you like the change in yourself very much.

> It changes your personality. It changes you. I think it's made me much more tolerant. And certainly able to empathize with people more.

You will be much less uptight about everything. We said there was no "solution" to the "Suitcase Problems," but there is, is one sense. You can outgrow them. And that is what being a cardiac couple comes down to. Living a life that makes both of you happy, a life that makes sense to both of you. His heart attack is not a handicap, it is an opportunity. It forcibly stripped away from both his and your eyes a lot of assumptions about how you "had" to live and what it takes to make you happy. But it managed that without making the knowledge useless. There is no physical fact about his condition that must now stand in the way of your reconstructing a better life than you would have had without the attack. None. Including the threat of other heart attacks.

Take it from this Heart Wife. Her husband had a number of attacks and finally died, fourteen years after the first one. But until then . . . oh, how he lived!

> My husband said that he felt the fourteen years during the time he had his coronary condition were the happiest years of his life.
>
> And he was a very content man—he had an interesting, stimulating, and satisfying life.
>
> I always felt this was quite a compliment to the way it worked out and the way we all handled it, that he found these years the most satisfactory.

We reevaluated many of the things that we had been doing. And in reevaluating them we were able, perhaps, to concentrate on the things that were really important to us as a family.

People would say to me, "You really haven't had very good luck!"

But I really feel it's not what happens but what you do about what's happened to you that makes the difference.

If you know what your goals are, it's a little easier to keep going in the right direction. And we treasured many things.

We had a very wonderful life!

It is a different life. But it can be a wonderful difference, a wonderful life. You do give up things, but for the most part they are things that brought you scant pleasure before. You give up a little to get a lot, including a closer, richer relationship with your husband. Five years from now, if someone asks you what kind of life you are leading as a cardiac couple, you will wonder, "Compared to what?" Because it will be hard for you to imagine that you could ever have been leading another kind.

CHAPTER

16

Prophets and Loss

"Self-fulfilling prophecy" is a very handy concept, one that offers insight into many puzzling human relationships. Including the way a Heart Wife, if she is not careful, can help make an invalid of her husband—a "cardiac cripple."

The premise of the self-fulfilling prophecy is that you make things happen by saying they will happen. It is not magic; it is the simplest sort of common-sense psychology. In sports it is called "psyching your opponents," convincing them they are so overmatched (by peerless you), they might as well not bother trying. Once they believe it and start telling themselves the same thing—in effect, prophesying their own defeat—they do not play to win. Why bother? So they lose, and the prophecy has fulfilled itself.

You can "psych" yourself, as well. By prophesying your own victory, you can become convinced you are a winner—which makes you go out on the tennis court or golf course and "play over your head," beating someone who is actually better than you.

A self-fulfilling prophecy does not have to be spoken. It can be an action, like a faith healer's laying-on of hands. If the belief is strong enough, the prophecy of recovery becomes self-fulfilling, especially with diseases born in, or complicated by, the mind. That is why self-fulfilling prophecies sometimes seem to work miracles.

But they are not always constructive.

They can also convince a person that the very worst is about the best he can expect. When the prophecy—in words or action—is that a patient will not recover, will not get his strength back, will not lead a happy, normal life, it can make the patient, if he believes it, give up hope and give up trying.

Ask any doctor about "the will to live."

The way you treat your husband can have a direct bearing on how quickly and completely he gets over the effects of his coronary. Because the way you treat your husband is, in effect, your prophecy about how his recovery will go and what its outcome will be.

He came home an invalid. If you continue to treat him like an invalid, if you act as though he cannot do anything for himself, you are prophesying chronic invalidism for him.

What *is* treating him like an invalid? Roughly, everything you do or say that proceeds from the assumption that he is an invalid, continuing to do things for him long after he should be doing them himself.

And yet it is so *hard* not to treat your husband—some ways, some of the time—as though he were an invalid. You love him. You are anxious to make things easy for him, to take care of him. It comes naturally to a wife to want to do things for her husband, all the more so when he is sick! When he first comes home, it is necessary. The line, after all, is drawn at doing for him what he cannot do for himself; but that line keeps changing as he grows stronger, and no one is smart enough to chart it's exact position day by day or even week by week.

Mercifully, you have a lot of leeway. One inopportunely changed light bulb may make a scene, but it does not make a prophecy. In fact, any given number of wrong things done and wrong things said do not make a prophecy. Furthermore, nothing you do or say will turn him into an invalid if he is determined not to be. A prophecy cannot be self-fulfilling if it is not believed.

Then what is all the fuss about?

Well, most men are not so adamantly sure they will recover. A fair proportion of them start off more than half convinced they will not. In either case, what you do can tip the balance.

Take meals as an illustration. Let's say that the first week home, he is supposed to have his meals in bed. Comes the second week, and he is "too tired" to get up for them. What are you going to do—let him starve? So you continue to bring him his meals in bed. Through no conscious plan of your own, you are acting as though he is, indeed, an invalid who *must* have meals in bed because he is too weak to get up. What you do, in turn, reinforces his self-image as an invalid, making it harder for him to get up. And round-and-round we go.

That is one way you can "help" him become a cardiac cripple. An even more common way—we all are prone to act and speak like this, now and then—is the worried "Are you sure it's all right for you to . . ."—with practically anything ending the sentence. Say it often enough, about enough activities and he will start to wonder if, as a matter of fact, it *is* all right. And the man who gets into the habit of anxiously wondering if it is all right for him to be increasingly active is well on his way back to bed. To stay.

Do Heart Wives really say things like that? Of course! Because we are worried and we do wonder. What's more, there are occasions (especially at first) when a firm, declarative "You know you are *not* supposed to be doing that" is more in order than a question. It is not the phrase but the attitude that is the problem.

Here are two contrasting attitudes, given to us by two different Heart Wives. Interestingly enough, they use the same illustration:

> When I'd take a shower, it was always with the door open, in case—you know, I wouldn't hear if he needed something, or something was wrong and he called.

Now the second Heart Wife:

It's very, very aggravating to a man—especially when he's
sick and he knows it—for you to be always saying, "I'm going
here, I have to do this or that, I'm going to take a shower; if you
want me, you yell."

It's constantly reminding him of his incapacity. "You can't do
it yourself, I have to do it for you," is what you're saying.

It's one of the worst things you can do.

One of the Heart Wives who urged this point on us most
forcefully knows what it is like from the patient's side of the
bed. She had a critical illness not long before her husband's heart
attack. She said:

Some men become "cardiac cripples"—and ofttimes their
families help them become one.

The fact that I was so sick helped me to understand about not
holding back and not "mothering" him. Because I resented it
when I was down, if there was a gasp of worry any time I turned
over.

Your apprehensions will increase his apprehensions.

She knows from her own annoyance how easy it is to feel, not
helped and comforted, but smothered by cloying oversolici-
tousness.

One husband put it a little differently at a post-hospital
meeting. We had complimented him on his unrelenting cheer-
fulness and patient determination not to let his heart condition
matter. He replied:

Listen—if I didn't get up and going, I could just sit around and
let my darling wife be my darling wife and wait on me hand and
foot. And she would gladly do it! Nothing's too much for her!

But if I let her—okay, I might as well crawl into a wheelchair
and have a sign on my neck, "I am an invalid."

A different case shows what can happen when a Heart Wife,
out of her apprehension and eagerness to do everything she can
for her husband, does too much. The case is so much to the
point, so pat, it almost appears that anxieties on your part

instantly communicate themselves to your husband and relentlessly march both of you into a permanent invalid-suite for two. That is not the way it happens, of course. As with most human relations, things do not follow one another with such nice precision. And we do not mean to get you tense and anxious about each slight nag, every random bit of hovering. It is not the end of the world, or the end of his recovery.

Still, a thoroughgoing anxiety on your part, an implacable mothering attitude, can take on the aspects of a self-fulfilling prophecy. It certainly did in the case of Mr. H—as shown in the following notes we made after each contact with his wife:

Today was the second meeting for these Heart Wives. . . .

Mrs. H's husband will have a pacemaker inserted tomorrow, and she's quite apprehensive. She kept asking if the doctors would give her instructions on how to care for her husband and what to do if there was a sudden problem. She left the meeting several times to go and check on her husband. . . .

[ten days later]

Spoke to Mrs. H on the telephone today. Her husband has been home three days, and she says he is very weak—unable to feed himself or walk or even get himself out of bed. First time he tried he fell to the floor, and she ran screaming to the apartment next door for help. She said it would have been better if he had stayed in the hospital an extra week until he had gathered more strength. . . .

[three days later]

Mrs. H called Friday, on the verge of hysteria. She kept repeating that the hospital should have kept her husband another week (at least) or until he could at least walk by himself to the bathroom and be self-sufficient. She cried that she was exhausted and could not go on carrying him to the bathroom and being on twenty-four-hour duty at home. She had called his doctor to tell him it wasn't "working out." The doctor decided he would be better off at a rest home, and was going to send an ambulance to their apartment. . . .

[next day]

Mrs. H called from the hospital to say that the rest home had *not* given Mr. H the proper care. In fact, they had forgotten to give him his necessary medicine, which was a great source of worry to both of them. . . .

Mrs. H drove to the doctor's office, determined to change the situation. The doctor apparently received her very warmly and reassured her. Mr. H was readmitted to the hospital for further medical care and treatment.

Mrs. H is greatly relieved and thankful. She repeated several times what a nice room he had and what great attention he was getting in the few hours that he had already been there. She was very hopeful that he would gain strength there and be home only when he was strong enough to take care of himself. . . .

[two days later]

I visited Mr. H. He is a very quiet man normally, and now (Mrs. H has told me) he only speaks in a whisper. After a while, Mrs. H asked if it was all right if she went down to the fourth floor with me to see some of her "old friends" from the previous week.

On the way down she said how terrible it was for him to have gone home when he was unable to walk and eat. She said he wet his bed because he was unable to get to the bathroom. She had to take him all his meals in bed. For all these problems, she looked very well. I was happy to see this.

After Mrs. H returned to her husband's room, the nurse who had been taking care of Mr. H when he was here before said she had spent over an hour talking to him that morning.

She said that apparently he was doing fairly well until he went home. He was talking clearly, and the doctor's exam showed no reason he could not now. According to nurses on the floor and the attending doctor, he *was* walking in the hospital. Mrs. H insists he could only walk if he was leaning heavily on her.

There are almost unlimited occasions, especially during the initial weeks after your husband comes home, when you are sorely tempted to invite your husband "to lean heavily on you," to become a nursemaid, to mother him. If you give in to the temptations, it is a two-way prophecy. The more you become a nursemaid and mother to him, the more he will need that kind of support and care. And the more you will *become* a nursemaid and mother to your husband—and cease to be a wife.

The period of actual, medical-physical dependency, when he does need some nursing, even mothering, ends quite soon. Then you must let go just as steadily and rapidly as possible. As one Heart Wife put it, you must "let out the tether." She went on to compare the process with raising children. And insofar as your husband starts off needing a measure of mothering, that is a pretty accurate analogy.

> When he was getting well, it's just like when your kid learns to drive.
>
> He was no longer with me; he was taking the car, being on the freeways, being out of my sight all day. And I was anxious—but I don't think I showed him my apprehension.
>
> I had to make a lot of changes in my way of looking at things. I had to let go of him, let him be a man and get well.
>
> I had to stop hovering.

Hovering. That one word says volumes about the creation of cardiac cripples. In the early stages of recovery it conjures up a picture of a nervous wife lurking just outside the bedroom door, waiting for any sound that might suggest her husband needs something, from a glass of water to an ambulance. The atmosphere is heavy with the apprehensive prophecy of chronic, helpless invalidism.

Later on, hovering is more subtle, but less destructive only in that the husband has already set foot firmly on one path or another: back to the world—or back to bed.

At all stages, the self-fulfilling prophecy can be just as powerful a positive force as it can be negative.

The difference is not in specific actions. It is the spirit of your actions, not the actions themselves, that makes the wheels go 'round in the effect you have on your husband during his recovery. Of course, he needs to be "taken care of," as one of the psychiatrists we talked to said, freely, gladly, and unstintingly. He needs to be shown he is treasured and wanted. But as a husband, not as a child.

A husband we'll call Mr. L is a case in point. Following his second heart attack he said he was eager to get well, to get out of the house and back to work. After the first attack, he had spent almost eighteen months at home, reversing roles with his wife almost completely. She got a job; he did the housework, cooking, looking after the kids. He realized it had prolonged his feelings of impotence and probably recovery, and was determined not to let it happen again.

Mr. L did not mention what role his wife had played, or had not played, in deciding the nearly disastrous course of his first recovery. In fact, he did not mention his wife at all. And we had the clear impression that she no longer played a very large part in his thoughts or plans. He did not seem to feel that she mattered or was a factor to reckon with in his plan for recovery or for living. He was not blaming her for what had happened before. At least not at that meeting (which would have been an unlikely place for such unburdenings). But there was a clear implication that, since she had not done anything to help before, she was not going to get an opportunity to help or hinder now.

That is a sad situation for both of them as a married couple. It is also a sad situation for him as a recovering heart patient.

Long after the time when a man is as totally recovered as he will ever be from a heart attack, his wife will have to help him cope with what seems to be a universal tendency of men with heart conditions, almost like a reaction to the earlier danger of becoming cardiac cripples: they become impatient with the permanence of a heart condition. In short, they act like children. Some sooner, some later. But sooner or later, all of the men we have met or have been told about by their wives become childish about the rules.

As we said in the first chapter, the permanence of a heart condition and the consequent need to observe some rules is what distinguishes heart attacks from most diseases. Living through a heart attack is not difficult; the hard part is living with a heart attack. Forever.

But that is just what your husband must do. No crash diets for him, no fits and starts of exercise, no "catching up on lost sleep" or taking a long weekend to recover from the murderous last week. It is regular food, exercise, rest, and diminished strain—or else!

Or else what?

No one is sure. He must be content to know that the best medical opinion is that he materially improves his chances by following the rules.

Men get tired of this routine. Sometimes it happens almost at once, more often it is after a number of trouble-free years. They act like children in their "defiance" of the doctor, nature, and you. Because they are anxious to prove they are not children but men, the most usual form of defiance, early in recovery, is rushing back to work. Later on, the usual acts of defiance are:

— ignoring pain or other warnings to slow down;

— resisting diet;

— lifting, rushing, "showing off," displaying stamina or toughness;

— in general, overdoing.

What can you do about any of these or any like them?

What you should not do is treat him like a child simply because he is acting like one. You *know* what that will do: make him all the more childishly defiant. You cannot treat your husband like a child and expect him to respond in anything other than a destructive way. On the other hand, you can skirt the issue by doing exactly what you feel must be done to protect him from stresses or temptations that seem clearly harmful, but doing it in a way that gives him every opportunity to see it as something other than unwarranted interference on your part, to accept it—and you—in the best possible way. But remember, however adept you become in that technique of artful intervention, do not mistake it for a good thing. The goal is adjustment and an automatic "cardiac couple" life-style; no amount of intervention on your part, be it ever so tactful, is a positive good.

It never advances the cause of adjustment. It is always an emergency measure.

Remember that different people have different needs. Some men simply cannot give up certain activities that ideally should be curtailed. The deprivation would make them more fretful and make their adjustment to other aspects of a sensible life-style that much harder. One Heart Wife told us about her reactions to what, objectively speaking, was ruinous activity for a man who had suffered a heart attack. But it is hard not to agree with her conclusion that interference on her part would have been much worse.

MRS. G: He was given a promotion at work at the beginning of last year. And he was very happy about that. You know, he felt he had reached what he had strived for for so many years.

He devoted a tremendous amount of time to working—and I was uneasy about the amount of time he was spending at work.

H.W.C.: Because his promotion required more responsibility?

MRS. G: Well, it required more responsibility—but, then, he became a victim of circumstances. It just so happened, with the industry he's in, that there were a lot of things that took place. It is the steel business—and there was a steel strike pending, and there was the harbor tie-up, and just a whole lot of things that required a lot of thought.

And he was working, I'd say, close to twelve hours a day. But he seemed to be enjoying it so much, as a wife you can't help but wonder—well, if someone is enjoying something so much, can it really be bad for him?

I don't remember a time when he ever enjoyed working as much as he did then.

Even if it is not so terribly important to him, sooner or later you will have to let him do it. You are not a nursemaid, nor his mother. He is an adult, no matter how childishly he acts now and then. If it is not something that obviously is going to be a serious, damaging experience, just forget it. As we said before, a little egg yolk won't kill him, a lot of fussing might. More probably, what it will kill is your marriage—or hopes of fine, future adjustment. And more to the point, if you keep nagging him not to do things that are important to him, you will convince him he's an invalid.

If Jane can watch Arthur lift a couple of cinder blocks into place for a bookshelf without saying a word (strangled cries, followed by the faint sound of some very expensive orthodontia being ground to bits doesn't count), if JoAnn can watch Forrest rush out to an occasional late-night meeting with a paranoid client without saying a word (well, maybe one—but it's very short, only four letters, and he is gone by then anyway)—if we can, then you can too!

Many years after there is even the remotest possibility of your husband becoming a cardiac cripple, there will still be a lively chance of *your* becoming a "cardiac widow"—like the wife of Mr. L, who no longer figured in his plans.

That can happen, for a slightly different reason, to the Heart Wife who becomes a nag. What can you do about your husband's excesses but nag? Mrs. S gave us, if not an answer, at least a direction for our thoughts:

MRS. S: At times I hear myself as a nag and a picker. And then I think to myself, "What is worse? He's going to do what he wants to do anyway. And he's going to react negatively to my picking and nagging. So you may as well shut up!"

But sometimes when you're sitting down to have a drink together, you can say, "As a human being, and as your wife, I am really concerned. It worries me and makes me upset. I would feel better if you, you know, if you didn't smoke so much, or you didn't overeat, or you didn't do this or that. I'm just telling you how I feel."

H.W.C.: You pick the right moment and the right setting for calm, non-"arguey" words.

Mrs. S: Right. But I feel that when you're constantly uptight, and giving ... *directions,* orders—*"don't* smoke; *don't* overeat; *don't* eat that, there's too much fat in it; *don't* touch the liver pâté"—you do get to sound like a real nag. And I think that turns people off.

H.W.C.: I agree. A lot of wives act this way, and they don't like themselves for it. But they say, "Well, what can I do differently?"

Mrs. S: Well, other people are appalled by me. Like our partner's wife said, *"Well!* can't you stop your husband from smoking? I am *surprised!"*

And I just say, "He's a big boy, and I am not his mother. I don't want him to smoke, and he knows he shouldn't smoke, and there's nothing more I can do."

He knows how I feel about it. But to go out for an evening and keep saying, "Don't smoke, don't do this, don't eat an egg." I mean, I can't do it—I won't do it! I'm really not his mother!

H.W.C.: I don't think he wants you to be.

Mrs. S: No! He really doesn't. And it's his life, it's his body. And it's his responsibility. And I've said to him, "Lookit, your kids still need you, and I need you. And we really want you to be here—and it doesn't look like you're trying very hard."

H.W.C.: When you say that, what does he say to that?

Mrs. S: He doesn't answer.

Of course not. It was a silly question for us to have asked. What can a man in those circumstances answer? There are no appropriate words. There are, however, two appropriate actions: he can think about what his wife said, and realize what he has been doing and stop doing it; or he can decide that he is so fed up with the necessary restraints on him that he will ignore them and take his chances. If this choice is presented to him the tenth year after his heart attack, what he decides will be hugely influenced by how his wife has made him feel about her and his cardiac life-style during the preceding nine years. If it has been a question of continual nagging, reproaches, and interference, he will be much less disposed to a reasonable decision.

As we said, it is not easy to be still when you see your husband doing things you know are silly acts of childish defiance against, well, Fate is probably the closest. But it is essential that you try. That you don't hover.

If you are not sure you can manage, we offer the JoAnn and Jane Emergency Temptation Kit: Everytime he starts "proving himself" to the world, and most especially you, showing that he is perfectly all right, every bit the man he used to be, whenever he stays up too late or exercises too much or eats something on the no-no list—in short, when he acts like a child—take a napkin, or any square of cloth, fold it into the familiar triangle shape, and tie it firmly over *your* mouth.

If it happens too often and the excesses are too great, choose your moment and talk to him "as a human being and as a wife." Not as a nag, mother, or scold.

The parting thought comes from a Heart Wife who was explaining why she had insisted her husband keep track of his own medication, even though he had always been very absent-minded about such things:

> I found myself nagging, "Did you take your pills, did ya take your pills? dijatakeyrpills?"
>
> I didn't want to. I was getting to feel like a nagging mother about those goddamn pills. And I like our love affair too much to be that!

Which brings us to the agreeable subject of our next chapter.

CHAPTER

17

This Marriage Is Still Rated "X"!

The most important thing that can be said on the subject of sex in the lives of coronary patients was said to us by Dr. Reuben Koller, one of the few psychologists in the country who specializes in the sexual problems of heart patients: *A heart attack has absolutely no physiological effect on a man's sexual ability.* No matter what the songs and stories say, "affairs of the heart" have only the slightest connection with the heart. Physiologically, that is.

The *psychological* effect of a heart attack on a man's sex life is a different matter. A heart attack can have a considerable effect on how a man thinks about sex; and that can be disabling as far as performance goes. But there is no physical reason it should be so. And the purpose of this chapter is to help you make sure that in your husband's case it will not be.

First of all you have to see clearly what the problems may be and how they come about. Despite the number of experiences we heard from Heart Wives—and, of course, our own experiences—we did not see the problems of postcoronary sex very clearly or as a coherent whole until our series of conversations with Dr. Koller. We have come to see that the problems so many couples experience with sex after a heart attack involve a total intertwining of what the husband fears, and why, what he is trying to prove, and what the wife does to protect him and their marriage.

Because the problems are psychological, some fairly weird things can happen. But only along one of two lines. Husbands become something of satyrs, or somewhat impotent. We will look at the satyrs first.

The Temporary Satyr

As Heart Wives told us their experiences we were struck by the curious fact that husbands who came home from the hospital acting like satyrs never stayed that way for long. One Heart Wife put it this way:

> I was very frustrated with the sexual situation for a reason I didn't expect.
>
> My husband seemed to be more interested than usual. He was trying to prove something to himself, and I didn't know how to handle that situation.
>
> I went to talk to the doctor, but he just sort of tossed it off casually. And I guess I decided, well, the doctor wasn't that concerned, so I must be wrong to be worried.
>
> Anyway, things just got back to normal by themselves. We got back into our old patterns and that was that. It was a temporary thing.

Another Heart Wife said that the only word for her husband's attitude about sex, once the doctor said it was all right to resume intercourse, was "uncontrollable." She also felt her husband was having to prove himself, but to her as much as to himself. He insisted on having intercourse almost every night, although before the attack, she said, it had been "when the spirit moved them." And he seemed especially anxious about her reaction; he kept asking her during, immediately after, and between times, whether she enjoyed sex as much as before. She felt the sexual situation was related to her husband's insistence on returning to the same work he had been doing before the attack, which involved more physical labor than she thought was good for him. It seemed to her that she could not say anything to him about sex because it would be a put-down to his virility. The fact was that his new, heightened level of sexual activity was anything but satisfying to her; it was frightening! And he flatly refused to discuss the possibility of another line of work.

Not knowing what to do, she did nothing. Yet, within six months their sex life had returned to normal. And he had gotten another job.

When we mentioned these cases to Dr. Koller, he was not at all surprised. He outlined the general course of this kind of reaction, starting in the hospital:

> While the patient is still in the hospital, still shaken up by the attack, he doesn't even have sexual fantasies.
>
> But once he knows that he's not dead, or dying, there's a sort of sexual recovery. Nurses become extremely appealing, even nurses that might be less than appealing on the street, just because they're female.
>
> It's not uncommon for a patient to have erections during certain activities, like when a nurse bathes him. This can be disconcerting, to both of them. Like, there it is! Surprise! But it's also very gratifying to the patient. That he is *able* to have an erection.

Gratifying, but not enough. Now he knows he can, but he still does not know if it makes the slightest difference. Maybe nobody cares! Dr. Koller went on to point out:

> It's not unheard of for a man at certain age milestones to wonder "How attractive am I to women? How much of a man am I still?"
>
> Well, a heart attack is certainly more of a blow than passing an age milestone!
>
> He may say, "Hey, wait a minute! Is it still possible for a woman to want me—even though I might be an invalid?"
>
> In my experience, that stops of its own accord, especially if he's given some support, if he's treated normally, not like an

invalid. He's trying to see how attractive he is, particularly to his wife. It is not a sign that he's going to be adulterous.

In fact, the sort of overinterest in sex we are talking about is almost the opposite of adultery. What the man is trying to prove to himself and to his wife is best proven in bed with her, not in clandestine motels.

But there never really was any reason for him to have worried about his masculinity (remember what Dr. Koller said at the start: a heart attack will not interfere, physically, with a man's sex life). Once the sudden satyr finds out that he has not been sexually disabled, or even impeded, by his heart attack it is no longer necessary to prove anything to anyone. His "overinterest" in sex quickly subsides to whatever level it was at before the attack. It is that simple.

Impotence

Unfortunately, the other problem is not so simple. According to Dr. Koller—and the wide majority of Heart Wives we know—the problem most Heart Wives can expect to face is not a sudden burst of sexual athletics, but its opposite, impotence. Either the husband seems too apathetic to bother with sex, or too frightened of what he imagines may be the consequences to his heart even to try. Or, still worse, he does try—and meets with disastrous results.

At this point, a couple can find themselves in trouble. One Heart Wife told us:

> He just couldn't. We talked about it, and to the doctor. He was tested, and there was nothing wrong physically. He tried some medicine to help; but it didn't really seem to matter.
> We've just stopped trying now. I stopped, that is. Because it was just making him feel worse and worse.

This sort of psychological impotence also starts in the hospital. Another Heart Wife said her husband showed signs, pretty early, that he saw even the mildest sexual arousal as a threat to his health and safety. She told us:

> The doctor had said something about "no sex for a while" when he was still in the hospital. And he was scared of his reaction.
>
> I went in to see him one day, and I put my hand under the blanket and touched him—as a joke. And he said, "Don't do that, for God's sake!"
>
> He really was nervous about that. "Don't do that, God! Don't do that!"

That degree of nervousness cannot be a very reassuring prelude for return to a normal sex life. Sure enough, when her husband got home:

> He was very uptight about intercourse. With all sorts of fears, checking himself, taking his pulse, and so on.
>
> I think a lot of the sensations he had—a closed-up throat and fluttering in the chest, or whatever—they were fear. So many fear symptoms are like symptoms of a heart attack.
>
> It took a couple of months to still his fear. But he never really got rid of it. Ever since he had his heart attack, we have not had sex as often.

How does it start?

Dr. Koller traced a typical psychological portrait of a man caught in what he termed a "spiral of impotence." Among the gloomy things the patient finds out in the hospital is that he will not be able to have sex for a while. And "be able" means two things. His heart is not up to it and he is not up to it. He knows it. He feels it. He may even be getting medication with side effects that make him literally, though temporarily, impotent. Then, when he is released from the hospital, his fear carries over to his view of the sexual aspect of his homecoming. Dr. Koller continued:

> If he thinks his wife will be making sexual demands on him that he may not be able to fulfill, it's just like his worry about "Will I be able to earn enough to support my family." It's the

same sort of thing. "Performance anxiety" is the term that is used.

Impotence is usually based on something like that. "I'm not going to be able to make it. Will she hate me when she realizes I can't do it? What'll happen to me—I'll be such a bad person, a failure."

And all this stuff makes him fulfill his greatest fear. He's *not* able to do it *because* he's anxious.

Anxiety, excitement—and happiness—have a lot of components that are similar, psychologically.

Our anxiety is based on telling ourselves how bad things are going to be. We react as though what's bad is happening right now.

For a patient to say, "I'm going to die when I have intercourse," is a kind of anxiety that could very easily lead to impotence. The part of the nervous system that deals with anxiety has to be shut down for sexual arousal to take place. An erection involves the part of the nervous system that is involved in sleeping. So if you're anxious, it's extremely difficult to get an erection. That's just the way our bodies are built.

If a man is anxious, frightened, his body is girded for fighting or running. It's not ready for sex. The result is impotence.

But "impotence" means a lot of things. It means you aren't able to get an erection. But it could also mean that you're no good, you have no strength, you're not a man, you aren't useful, you're use-*less*. All these things are hooked on to it.

It happens once and, "Uh-oh! It's all over: I'm going downhill."

Then the next time, you're more frightened, more anxious. And the next time, of course, you don't get your erection, either.

So both satyriasis and impotence start the same way. The patient is told he must restrict physical activity for a while. Including sex. But it is a matter of precaution, a question of "should he" or "shouldn't he," not can he or can't he. Although some of the medication he gets could inhibit erection, the patient does not know that. He thinks it is him—and his heart. At this point the two types of patient go their separate ways, depending on their individual personalities.

The satyr sets out to prove he is not impotent, as soon as he can, and by means of the most direct, obvious manifestation of his virility possible: intercourse with his wife, overdoing it because he *is* trying to prove himself. The impotent reacts to sex differently. He can feel what is happening! His heart, his breathing, the strain! How can that be safe when he is not supposed to exercise in other ways that might result in the same physical symptoms of strain? Are they trying to *kill* him—with love? Unlike the satyr, a man who finds frightening similarities between sex and the onset of a heart attack will never be able to "prove" to himself that what he fears is not so. Every time he starts making love to his wife, zing go the strings of his heart. And it sounds suspiciously to him like the funeral march. He gives up—or, at best, has sex cautiously, infrequently, nervously.

What You Know Can't Hurt You

The basic reason for fear about sex in heart patients is ignorance of what a heart attack means, sexually. And the basic treatment is to get rid of that ignorance. Dr. Koller put it like this:

> The key issue is to handle all the irrational fears, to get them out in the open and deal with them. Preferably while the patient is still in the hospital. And certainly with his wife there.
>
> You have to have them together, to have as many of their superstitions, as many of their anxious fantasies as possible grounded: "These things are *not* dangerous. *This* is not true; *that* is not true."

Specifically what is not true? Surprise! Practically everything your "common sense" tells you about Sex and the Heart Patient is wrong!

Here is what we were told by a Heart Wife who, if anything, was better informed than most of us are:

When my husband was ready to go back to work, we went
down to the doctor's office first. And we said, "How about sex?"

The doctor said, "Well, it's all right; but cautiously." Now
we have a joke about it: "How's your sex been lately—cautious?"

Which is funny—but *of course* it has to be cautious at first. I
wasn't exactly frightened, but I thought, "Sex is one thing he's
going to *feel.*" They put everything into it, you're using every
muscle in your body. Your heart is pounding—and you can't
help thinking, "What's going to happen?"

Well, his heart does beat fast; he does start panting, perspir-
ing. Common sense tells you it is a strain on your husband's
heart. But the doctor must think it is not too much strain. Right?

Wrong. The doctor does not think it is any "strain"—at least
the way you mean it. It is *not* bad for the heart, lungs, and
circulatory system to be doing what they are doing, while your
husband and you are doing what you are doing. The question is
not whether the doctor is right about whether your husband's
heart is well enough to take the strain your common sense tells
you is put on it; the question is, "How much strain *is* it, really?"
And the answer is: much, *much* less than you think it is, and
nothing like what the physical symptoms make it appear.

To quote Dr. Koller:

> When the patient gets out of the hospital, the doctor knows
> what he is capable of doing. Can he run around the block? Or
> should he walk around the block? Can he climb a flight of stairs,
> can he climb two, three flights of stairs? Can he go back to work?
> Can he lift? How much can he lift? All this is worked out.
>
> Well, for the typical patient—a middle-class, middle-aged,
> long-married man—sexual activity with his "wife-of-long-
> standing" is no more strenuous than climbing a flight of stairs or
> walking around the block. At a pretty brisk pace, but walking.
> In physiological terms, that's the strain it means.
>
> Now you have to look at it from the patient's viewpoint.
>
> What does he see when he thinks of sexual intercourse, or
> when he does it? Heavy breathing. Perspiration. High heart
> rate. Sometimes gasping for breath. *But*—if he can do the ac-
> tivities I mentioned, he can have sex. Because the kind of stress

that is involved in intercourse is very short-lived. There's a sudden peaking at ejaculation, and a sudden dropping. So, yes, you get this relatively intense physiological activity, but it won't be for any length of time.

The doctor knows how much strain he can take. Well, if he can take any of the strains I mentioned, he can take sex, most certainly.

All this is predicated on the physiological capacity of the patient. And that can only be determined by the individual patient's doctor.

But, as a guideline, sexual activity of the average married man is no more stressful than walking around the block a couple of times—and that's not very much. It's certainly nothing like running a hundred-yard dash, which is the way a lot of patients see it.

But, you see, that's the idea: information allows a patient to re-label, allows him to say, "That is *not* a frightening thing."

You *do* see, don't you? There is an enormous difference between saying, "That is not a frightening thing" because it is no more of a strain than a walk around the block—and what your "common sense" tells you: "The doctor thinks my heart is healed enough to stand what must be a terrific strain."

Dr. Koller is not just guessing about the physiological strain of sex. In collaboration with three colleagues, Drs. Kennedy, Butler, and Wagner, he published an article called "Counseling the Coronary Patient on Sexual Activity," in the April 1972 issue of *Postgraduate Medicine*. It included the results of laboratory studies made on the effect of intercourse on heart rate and blood pressure. To quote from the article:

They studied 48 post-coronary subjects and 43 normal, coronary-prone subjects to determine the differential effects of sexual activity and other daily activity. Data were obtained at six-month and yearly intervals. . . .

The conclusion was that the physiologic cost of sexual activity is modest for middle-aged, middle-class, long-married men, especially in comparison with young volunteers in laboratory settings. In patients monitored during coitus, heart-rate response to sexual activity was minimal. . . .

These heart-rate responses are similar to those observed in the same individuals during regular daily activity such as driving a car, discussing business, or climbing one or two flights of stairs.

What Can You Do?

First of all you can banish "common sense" from your mind. Because what you think and feel about sex is bound to affect your husband. As one Heart Wife said to us:

About six weeks after Ron got home, the doctor said it was okay to go ahead. But after the first time, I was too frightened. I'd have rather waited six months than take a chance or keep on doing it that way—like, "How are you? You have a pain?"
You know?

Another Heart Wife said:

I remember feeling his heart. It was pounding, about a mile-a-minute, and then I would get worried.
It was really lousy! And I was always conscious, for months after, about his heart beating fast.

Fears like that can make sexual readjustment almost impossible for both husband and wife. As another Heart Wife put it,

They may not know it, but wives show their worry every single minute of the day. And if their husbands are aware of it, they are that much more uncomfortable.
They feel, "I'm not the man she married anymore. What good am I?"
I think the wife, knowing how he feels, must be careful not to seem apprehensive or scared. Especially in sex, the slightest sign that she is not accepting everything fully in the same way she always has can really be crushing.
If she holds back, if she says, "Honey, maybe you shouldn't do this," or, "Honey, don't you think that we should stop now?" that's the worst possible thing she can do. And right at that

moment could be the worst time of his life. And for their future life together.

One trouble is that many Heart Wives mistake the nature of their responsibility, assuming that it is medical as well as marital. They start wondering whether the doctor really *knows*. Well, no one can help wondering. But to decide the doctor does not really know, and what's more, that you know better, is foolish.

Remember, from the doctor's point of view, your presence in "his case" is mere accident. The point came up in our discussion with Dr. Koller when we asked:

> How can you stop from worrying when you feel your husband's heart racing and all that? When he's in the hospital, the hospital's taking care of him. When he's home, you're in charge.

Dr. Koller replied:

> Exactly! The point is they wouldn't send him home if they felt there was a real risk. The doctor is not going to look to the wife to act as a coronary-care nurse; and that's one of the first things a wife should be told, "Do you think the doctor considers you a coronary-care nurse? Do you have the kind of training where you would know if something bad is about to happen? Of course not! So if there were any real risk, we'd keep him right here."
>
> They're not going to trust his life to someone who isn't trained to look for the signs if they thought there was any *need* to look for signs.

How does the doctor know it's okay for your husband to resume sexual activity? Simple. He hinges his decision on various objective signs of overall returning strength, then establishes conditions to make sure any sexual activity is well inside the limits he knows your husband can take.

For instance, we discussed the sexual aspects of postcoronary recovery with Dr. Selwyn Bleifer, a cardiologist who makes it a point to keep up with researches in sexual physiology. Stressing the importance doctors put on sticking to what (and whom) you are used to, he began with a fairly funny line. He said, "When

a patient asks me if it's okay to start having sex, I tell him sure,
go ahead. But make sure it's with your wife. I don't want you to
get too excited." He immediately explained why.

This must be the original cardiological joke on the subject;
over half the Heart Wives we know have been told a variation
on the joke, greeting it with degrees of indignation ranging
from great to enormous. Very few were told the reason, even
necessity, behind the thought, if not the joke.

As Dr. Koller put it, when we mentioned the situation to
him:

> Well, it would be nice if all doctors explained what they
> meant, the principle behind it, the way the doctor you talked to
> did. It is very important.
>
> An extramarital affair could be dangerous for a heart patient.
> It could be as physiologically strenuous as sex is for a man who
> has just been married. And, for a newly wed, the amount of total
> bodily strain goes even higher than with premarital sex.
>
> After you're married a while, there's a tapering-off of stress.
> And it stays at a level for most of the rest of the marriage.
>
> It's a matter of habituation. That's not to say there is no kick.
> But it is stabilized at a lower level. That's the way our bodies
> react to anything new or exciting. After a while the newness,
> the excitement, wears off.

The doctor guards against undue stress in his instructions. One
Heart Wife told us:

> The doctor said something like, "Don't do it for six weeks.
> And when you start in, again, you can have intercourse, but
> don't do it hanging from the chandelier. No acrobatics."

Different doctors set different standards. One pegged a return to sex to the husband's ability to walk a certain distance.
The Heart Wife said:

> Each time my husband would walk a little further, and the
> doctor would say, "Any pain?"
> "No."

"Okay, walk a little further."

And he'd walk a little further—and he kept saying, "Okay, *when*, doctor?"

"Well, when you walk twelve blocks—a mile."

So my husband tells this joke, he says, "I immediately ran out and walked twelve blocks—and then I was too tired!"

The joking to one side, why twelve blocks? As we have learned, walking two blocks may put more strain on the heart than intercourse.

In effect, the other ten blocks are for safety's sake. The doctor knew that if the husband was strong enough to walk twelve, exertion equal to less than a two-block walk would have such a built-in margin of safety that sex could not possibly harm him. BUT THAT WAS NEVER EXPLAINED TO THE COUPLE.

So it would be totally understandable if they both became victims of "common sense" once they began intercourse. They would hear their own panting, feel their rapid heart beats, become aware of the perspiration—and begin to wonder if the doctor had correctly gauged how much strain was being put on the husband's heart.

Why aren't all cardiologists as quick as Dr. Bleifer was to explain their stamina tests and the limitations they prescribe? In their article, Dr. Koller and his colleagues gave this explanation:

Physicians, like other Americans, are often uncomfortable discussing sex. In addition, physicians usually have not been educated to deal with their patients' sexual difficulties.

The addition of comprehensive material about human sexual behavior to medical school curricula is changing this situation. However, many physicians have numerous pockets of misinformation or no information, and thus may hesitate to initiate discussion of the subject. The patients also tend to be restrained and, in addition, apprehensive. The result is that cardiac patients may receive little or inadequate assistance about sexual matters from their physicians.

And Dr. Koller commented to us:

> Why should an M.D. in cardiology be more aware of sex than some guy on the street? I don't mean medically. Of course, he knows medically, in general. But it is not his special field.
>
> He may very well feel it's intruding in his patients' private lives. So you have to bring it up.

The best thing to do is: MAKE SURE THE DOCTOR FULLY EXPLAINS IN EXPLICIT TERMS EXACTLY WHAT YOU AND YOUR HUSBAND CAN DO SEXUALLY AND WHAT THE EFFECT WILL BE ON HIS HEART.

As a guide to exactly how specific your questions should be, here is what Dr. Koller told us about the importance of demanding absolute frankness:

> Performance anxiety has to be dealt with before it happens. The husband has to be told—and his wife has to hear it—exactly what he can reasonably expect of himself. Knowing that—and knowing she knows—will lower his performance anxiety.
>
> He has to know just what positions and what circumstances are not risky. Because if he's afraid of dying or he's afraid of failing, those are both anxieties, and both are going to interfere with success.
>
> The doctor would tell him, "Don't expect, necessarily, to sustain intercourse long enough to give your wife an orgasm the first few times. You might get tired. Don't expect to do it husband-on-top; try it some other ways. If you want, try more foreplay, to bring your wife nearer to orgasm. And little by little you'll be able to stay in longer.

You want to know exactly what the doctor recommends for *you* and *your husband* (as opposed to some mythical "average couple") in the way of positions. You want to know, specifically, if any are ruled out, or are you and your husband perfectly free to experiment? Dr. Koller repeatedly pointed out to us that each case must be considered individually—and by the individual couple's own doctor. But he also pointed out the rich variety of experimentation possible:

The typical position, you know, is "male-on-top." But there are lots of others. For a patient who still has a lot of weight to lose, being on top would present a very difficult problem, because it is kind of a push-up that involves isometric exercise; and isometric exercise is dangerous for heart patients.

But with female-on-top, unless he tries to lift both of them off the bed, there's not that much risk. And side-by-side's not bad; and rear entry is certainly one of the least strenuous positions for the male.

Also there's the whole area of experimentation with foreplay and stimulation on both sides. None of that is even particularly stressful, certainly nothing like ejaculation or orgasm during intercourse.

It is all part of what you should ask the doctor. If he says no sex for X number of weeks, or until your husband has walked a certain distance, or whatever, find out exactly what he means by "no." Is kissing all right? How much and how long and where must it stop? How about "petting" (and where)? Is it all right for you to induce orgasm without intercourse through oral sex or masturbation? If not right away, when?

Of course, all that supposes you will be comfortable with whatever the doctor says is all right. Just do not be put off by any possible discomfort you think you may feel about *asking*. You may not be used to discussing these things with your husband (let alone someone else); the doctor may go into mild mid-Victorian shock (though we would bet against it). But which would you rather have—ten minutes of teen-ager embarrassment or months of anxiety? The question surely must answer itself. Because it certainly follows, no matter what your "common sense" tells you, that if you and your husband keep within whatever limits the doctor sets, you are this side of any plausible danger. And with apprehension out of the way, you can concentrate on fulfilling what is really your role, making what is really your essential contribution to your husband's recovery. Not as nurse, but as wife.

Your Role and Your Attitude

Discussions with the doctor make it easier for the Heart Wife and her husband. But they do not take away any of the need for a sympathetic attitude and compassionate response from the wife.

However, that is true regardless of heart attacks! It is not totally inconceivable that you had some sexual problems long before you ever dreamed of heart attacks. For instance, a frequent worry among new Heart Wives is the proper reaction on their part if they find they are not terribly well satisfied by their husbands at first (which, Dr. Koller suggested, is a distinct possibility).

Should a wife pretend orgasm to bolster her husband's confidence? Should she lie about it? We asked Dr. Koller. He made it clear that it is a question coming very close to one that can only be answered by therapy, which can only be given on an individual basis. But he did give us a sensible, general approach to the problem:

> It really is the same whether it's a question of a heart attack or not.
>
> She's worried about what will happen to their relationship: what he'll think of her, what happens to him, and his opinion of himself.
>
> Obviously he's interested in her satisfaction; and obviously he's hinging his own self-image on his performance. And he must have a lot of doubts about whether he's adequate or not.
>
> If he says, "Hey, did I satisfy you?" you can say, "Well, you know, it was pretty good; of course, I didn't have an orgasm because you didn't stay in long enough. But that's normal. That happens—just the way the doctor said it would. But I don't mind one bit! I'm willing to wait!"
>
> If he can't accept that, then they have to handle it with a professional.

That has to make sense for any woman who loves her husband and cares about his feelings. It even makes sense in the light of any experience you had before the heart attack, when something in your life as a couple, or his separate existence as an individual, had lacerated his confidence in himself. What did you do then?

Or turn it around. What did he do when you were in a reasonably similar position? During the latter stages of pregnancy, for example. It is a "dry period" for both of you, quite like now, except with roles reversed: then *you* could not; and he let you know he loved you and was waiting for the time when you *could* with happy anticipation and eager patience.

Now it is your turn.

Get that sense of anticipation across to him and it should go a long way toward quieting his trepidation. Especially if it is clear that you do not expect or need—and will feel no disappointment if you do not get—a display of sexual acrobatics (assuming, of course, you ever did). Besides, what does "satisfaction" mean? You have each other and are enjoying each other. Do there have to be skyrockets *every* time?

What is at stake is the long-run adjustment your husband makes to his entire coronary condition, to you as his wife, and to his life as half of a cardiac couple. It goes way beyond sex.

It means that in bed, as in other areas, you are not alone (so to speak). Nor should you be. Nor does his doctor, even if reticent about bringing up the subject of sex, want you to be.

After all, doctors are aware of the fact that the great psychological danger of a heart attack is neurotic anxiety, depression, and fear over a loss of manhood. Well, as everyone knows, sex is a powerful restorative for the spirits, a better relaxer than Miltown—and absolutely the single greatest reinforcer of masculine self-image and virility-confidence-inducer ever invented. It isn't bad fun, either.

CHAPTER
18

Divorce, Cardiac-style

You are reading this book because you love your husband and want to help him recover so you can both enjoy the golden fruits of a sunny marriage where, as the song said, every day is a holiday because you're married to me. Right?

Well . . .

Nearly one out of four marriages nowadays ends in divorce. Maybe you and he are separated, maybe you were about to be. Then came his heart attack, and you are not sure what to do. Call off the divorce? Postpone it? Go ahead? This chapter will help you sort out the possibilities and weigh the consequences of each.

The information in this book applies to you as much as to a happily married Heart Wife. You both face the same problems. You both will do the same things to help your husband's recovery. The difference is why you do them. She has a happy marriage and wants to keep it. You have a miserable marriage—and want a "happy" divorce, one leaving you emotionally free to start again. That makes your job harder than hers. Things will happen that are hard enough to put up with even for the sake of a happy marriage. For you, the unpleasant events will take place against the unpleasant background of an already failed marriage.

Still, it is worth the effort. If you can cope with the problems, you will walk away from the marriage with a free mind, an easy conscience, and clear emotions. Doing that is divorce, cardiac-style.

Or one kind, anyway. In all, there are five kinds of divorce, cardiac-style. We despise the first, fear the second, recommend the third—and hope you have the fourth or fifth.

You will find a chilling picture of the first kind in Eugene O'Neill's play *Mourning Becomes Electra*. In the Greek myth, when Agamemnon comes home from the Trojan War, his wife and her lover kill him. O'Neill set the story in New England at the end of the Civil War. His Agamemnon is a Union general in his fifties, married to a younger woman who loathes him and loves a sea captain.

General Ezra Mannon has a "weak heart." So, first, Christine tries "loving" him to death. No way! (Except maybe from surprised shock; he did not get much loving before he went off to war. But, as you know, cardiologists put sex right up there with Coumadin, Heparin, and polyunsaturates as a specific for heart patients.) Disgusted, but undaunted, Christine next tries something "sensible." She throws her infidelity in Ezra's face, rubbing it in with some details about her lover she knows will infuriate her husband the more. As she hopes, his rage brings on another angina attack, and that is her chance to switch poison for his usual medicine.

Poison aside, she demonstrates flawless technique. Who needs poison? It is messy, uncertain, detectable, and only marginally faster. By reversing everything we have discussed in this book, a woman should be able to generate enough tension, turmoil, and chaos to see her husband keel over inside of a month of leaving the CCU. That is the first kind of divorce, cardiac-style. The perfect (any way you look at it) crime: she has a truly *final* decree, without any tiresome wait; no lawyers to pay, property to divide, custody fights to settle; she gets everything—even sympathy!

Unthinkable? On the contrary. It is certainly unspeakable,

but it takes quite a bit of thought. It is the second kind that takes no thought. Our fear is that, unless you give almost constant thought to your position, you can easily let the relationship with your husband slip back into its old patterns of word and deed. Before, they led to your wanting a divorce; now they will relentlessly lead to the second kind of divorce, cardiac-style.

The only difference between this second kind and the first is intention, not result. Both can end with the husband in a rage—then back in the CCU, or his grave. But in the second kind the wife does not intend to provoke her husband's rage; she does not even mean to fight with him. She simply reacts, as usual, to his unreasonable behavior. She does not think of the consequences.

You are a Heart Wife. You have the key responsibility for establishing the atmosphere of recovery. But no atmosphere is created out of thin air; everything that went before must color it. And your feelings toward your husband hardly figure to be generous or kindly, given your plans for a divorce. Outrageous behavior that is merely the characteristic aftermath of a heart attack may seem, from him, just another page in the same old story. Without thinking, you may react to it the same old way, giving tit-for-tat what he gives you.

But this is a new story, with new complications. If the atmosphere of his recovery is envenomed by bitter quarrels and choking, heart-pounding rages—well, as we said, who needs poison? What will the result be if you have this kind of divorce?

In Chapter Four we discussed the guilt a woman often feels, even if she deeply loves her husband and is sure she did not consciously contribute to his heart attack. Unless you are devoid of human feelings, an emotional zombie, you already feel somewhat responsible for the original attack. If he has another now, while you are "in charge," you will know what part you played—and that knowledge will kill something in you.

All right, then, since it is so dangerous being part of his recovery, would you be smarter to go ahead with the divorce? It is a terrific temptation. Especially now, according to a psychiatrist who talked over the problem with us:

You see, to some degree every woman wants to get rid of her husband. And she wants to keep him. (The same is true of the husband, of course.) And I'm talking about completely "happy" marriages in which both partners want to stay married for life.

The reason is that everyone has faults. The most fervent lovers do and say things that annoy each other fairly often.

It's perfectly natural to want to get rid of faults. And just as natural to want to get rid of someone who annoys you. But if the fault belongs to the person you basically love and are married to, it's not so easy. In all likelihood, you can't get rid of the faults without getting rid of the person. In a "successful" marriage, you simply put up with the faults. Because the good points outweigh them.

In a marriage that is on the point of breakup, a heart attack can seem like just the latest and greatest of faults, the ultimate annoyance. Almost as if he did it on purpose. You'll resent the heart attack and think of it as some sort of dirty trick he's playing to upset your plans (in this case, for getting a divorce), just as he's always done.

One Heart Wife who was right on the edge of divorce when her husband had his heart attack, told us why she had called it off:

> What kind of woman does something like that? Walking out on a sick man! Why, they'd throw rocks at you!

Sure. And guess—just *guess*—who would cast the first! And the last. And, possibly, all those in between. You never need help throwing rocks at yourself; that is one target you never miss. If you leave him now, you give yourself maximum opportunity to feel guilty, no matter how things turn out. There are only two alternatives, both bleak.

You divorce him and he dies. Then how will you feel about the effect it had on his will to live? And what will your answer to that question do to you?

Or he gets well. If you have done nothing to help, how will you feel about yourself as a woman and wife? And what kind of shape will those feelings leave you in to be a woman and wife to someone else?

No matter how tough-minded you are, or think you are, can you honestly say that you could go on and make a new life without finding your self-reproaches emotionally and morally crippling? If so, good luck. If not, you should prepare yourself for the third kind of divorce, cardiac-style.

It means "standing by him"—not because he deserves it, but because you deserve a future free of guilt. How long must you stand by him? Until you know in your *own* heart that you have "done your duty." It's not a question of fooling him. If you were separated, there is no need to pretend that everything is fine now and that you are coming back (if he believes you, he is so far gone he probably will not last the night). If you were only discussing divorce, ignore the discussions; if he asks, tell him it is something you both must put aside for now; his getting well is important to both of you and your immediate concern is helping him do it.

It will not be easy. As we said, it is harder for you than for a Heart Wife who wants to continue her happy marriage to a man she loves. At least, she has that love to sustain her, and the promise of a happy future to reward her efforts. You have only the cold comfort of knowing it is not forever (something you should repeat to yourself about every hour) and the avid realization that when you are done with it, you can be done with him.

It is the difference between cooking a meal—and washing up afterward.

But at least when you get this third kind of divorce, cardiac-style, it will be with a clear slate and without shadows. The coronary was a bad break; but then, so was the marriage. Whoever promised you a rose garden?

Speaking of which, would you like a rose garden? Perhaps we can plant a couple of seeds of hope for you.

The fourth and fifth kinds of divorce, cardiac-style, are worth knowing about, watching, and hoping for.

If you are going to have the fourth kind of divorce, cardiac-style—you have unwittingly already had it; it happened when your husband's heart attack happened. To show you what we mean, let us tell you about a Heart Wife who had that kind of divorce.

For two years, Mrs. P watched her husband change into a bitter, narrow, miserably unhappy man. There was no explaining it, but her marriage seemed to be crumbling. Nothing she did seemed to make a particle of difference. Nothing she suggested—counseling, therapy, changes of job or neighborhood or state—nothing was "worth trying," because "nothing could possibly make a difference," according to her increasingly strange, and estranged, husband. Then, one night, she got a phone call.

> I heard "hospital" and I thought, "It's an accident." The way he'd been, I hated to have him drive. I was sure he was going to kill himself.
>
> When the intern said "heart attack," it was—well, almost a relief.
>
> I suddenly knew that's why he's been like that!

We have heard something like that from enough Heart Wives to make it a distinct possibility that it applies to you. Especially if your marriage problems became serious only a year or so before the attack, seemed inexplicable, and developed along lines like this:

Your husband changed. He became dissatisfied with practically everything, certainly with you. Even if you could get him to discuss it, he was not able to tell you anything that made sense. He did not point to specific things in you or in your marriage that were suddenly intolerable. It was just that everything was . . . wrong. You knew something was building up, some explosion. But you had resigned yourself to the idea that it was your marriage that was breaking apart.

Maybe not. Maybe it was his heart. The artery that eventually closed altogether was getting narrower, letting through less blood. So, even before the actual attack, his heart was operating under increasing strain, pumping blood with steadily decreasing efficiency. As his body got less blood, he began to have a generally rotten feeling that was almost guaranteed to taint his appreciation of everything. He felt stifled—quite literally, as well as figuratively, since with the diminished blood supply, his body was not getting enough oxygen.

Do you wonder that he was hostile and dissatisfied? Of course you expected something awful to happen: it *was* happening! Maybe you even found yourself hoping it would turn out to be . . . what? Well, *anything*—as long as that did not include the real and irreparable blowup between the two of you that you had about decided was inevitable.

When you heard "heart attack," did you suddenly, like Mrs. P, somehow "know" it would happen? If so, it may be that you have already had your divorce, cardiac-style. You will have to wait a while to be sure, but surely it is worth the wait!

The fifth kind of divorce, cardiac-style, takes even longer. But it, too, can save a marriage.

Can it save yours? That depends on why it was breaking up. If it was a general, growing dislike, or total lack of mutual interest—"incompatability" in its most real and personal (rather than merely legal) sense—then no, chances are your marriage cannot be saved, and most likely should not be. Divorce is the only remedy for true indifference.

But if there were certain, particular qualities (or lack of them), specific acts (or constant omissions) that made the marriage impossible, there is a chance. Especially if you know he still loves you and does not want you to go.

Just what was the problem? Can you give it a single, definite name? Infidelity? Overambition? Laziness? Irresponsibility? Those are some of the usual problems; and they all have the same basic cause. Immaturity. A childishly selfish attitude toward that great adult compromise called marriage.

Take the problem of infidelity. Maybe he can't help "lust-ing" after other women, but he *can* help chasing after them. He said he could when he said "I do." An adult says it and means it. He compromises, trading his "right" to go chasing for the benefits and comforts he expects from marriage. Men who aren't willing to make compromises like that are called bachelors. Men who say they will compromise, but who boyishly "have their fingers crossed," are called . . . well, let's settle for immature.

We are not talking about a man who runs off with another woman; in its own way that can be a perfectly mature (if finky) decision. We mean a man who wants what children want and what adults realize is not possible: to have his cake and eat it too.

That immaturity also shows up as unwillingness to face family responsibility in marriage. Like the "tycoon" who is so driven (and driving) he ends up giving his family *everything:* neuroses, insecurity, absentee love and care. And, finally, a short wait outside a Coronary Care Unit.

If your marriage was being destroyed by problems rooted in immaturity, you may find that his illness has "divorced" the problems from his personality, his life-style—or, hopefully, both. There is nothing like a heart attack, a stroke, or other serious illness for curing immaturity. It brings a man smack up against his own mortality and sets him thinking about what he really wants from life and what is really important in a life.

In some cases the exact, literal mechanics of the problem in the marriage may be "divorced" by the illness. Here's a case in point:

Mr. W was an avid sports fan and a fine athlete himself, having been a real star in school. When he married Mrs. W, he was spending most of every weekend playing golf—which she, basically uncoordinated, did not even play. And since she did consider herself a passable tennis player, she persuaded him to take it up, figuring they'd at least be together on the mixed-doubles court.

Within six months, he was so much better than she was that he became irritated at her incompetence whenever they played together. She soon gave up tennis. And three years later she was about to give him up:

I never saw him. He had season tickets to absolutely everything. That took care of most nights. Then every Saturday and Sunday he'd be off most of the day and be too beat when he did get back to do anything but flop down on the nearest chair and watch some damn football or baseball game on TV.

Ironically, Mr. W was sitting and reading when he had a massive coronary at the age of forty-four. The doctor told him light, rhythmic exercise, such as walking, was going to be his most strenuous "sport" for quite some time.

That degree of sports mania is clearly immature. But a heart attack has the "mechanical" effect of forcing a man to give up specific activities. He must try a new, more mature, life-style—at least for a while. Mrs. W thinks that her husband is developing enough new interests (including having her as a companion on prescribed walks) so that he will never again become wrapped up in sports to the exclusion of his family. But that really depends on whether the coronary has made him reevaluate his life and its priorities; it depends on just how much he has matured. In any case, though, their marriage now has a chance it never would have had otherwise. The coronary may mean that Mrs. W will get a fifth kind of divorce, cardiac-style—from the schoolboy sports-nut who was ruining her marriage to the *man* she loved.

The effects of heart attack in the next example are less obvious. No simple aspect of immaturity was the problem—just immaturity. But this case probably applies to many more people (except in its details, which are pretty lurid), just because the results *are* so undramatic.

Mrs. Y is about ten years older than her husband. After several years of marriage, they adopted a little boy. A few years after that, they separated; they had been apart for a little over two years when Mr. Y had a mild coronary at the age of thirty-five. She told us:

> After we adopted our son, things started to go sour for us. I knew I'd been babying my husband from the start. I guess it's what both of us wanted—with me older, it seemed natural; and

he liked it. But with a real baby around he couldn't feel like a man, letting me baby him too. And with the music industry near starving—it was too much for him to handle, so he started shooting-up heroin. With all that hassling—and me having a kind of alcohol problem on top of the rest—it wasn't any good anymore, and he couldn't take any more, so he just up and left.

Neither got a divorce, though. In fact, "We wanted to put our life back together, right along" as Mr. Y told us. But they had drifted too far apart to do anything about it. The shock of the coronary threw them together again. For the first time, both agreed to see a psychiatrist.

Both have deep problems, but now they both want to solve them. There may not be one visible cause (like Mr. W's sports-mania) that was mechanically eliminated by the illness. But enforced contemplation of life and its values made Mr. Y mature enough to realize how immature he had been. He says he wants a wife, not a mother; he wants to provide, not be provided for; he can accept Rudy as a son, not a rival.

Mrs. Y matured, too. She says that she has (in her own words) "outgrown playing with dolls"; she wants a husband, not a little-boy doll.

There is no way of knowing about either of these two marriages in the long run; but what marriage can you tell about for sure in the long run? The point is that in both cases—and maybe in yours, too—there is an unexpected happy side effect connected with your husband's coronary.

Divorce, cardiac-style, means making the very most of the very worst combination of events. And it means, at the very least, that you will survive in shape to start again.

CHAPTER
19

Have Your Egg Whites Sunny-side Up

It all depends on you. But then, it always did. You have always been the major influence in your family's eating habits. That does not mean you controlled everything they ate. There never was much you could do about your husband's lunch (even if you packed one for him); as for children—well, no one can fight pizza-power. Still, you were the main factor in shaping how your family thought about food, what general kinds of food they were accustomed to, the general style and content of the meals.

None of that has changed. But now your role, and the way you play it, has taken on vital importance for at least one member of the family. Your husband must adjust to a somewhat new way of eating. You still will not be able to control every bite he eats; you cannot make the adjustment for him any more than you can take his medication or his walks for him. But what you do and how you go about it can make all the difference in how quickly, thoroughly, and permanently he makes his own adjustment.

It all comes down to attitude. Yours will influence his. You can have him feeling what a sacrifice it is not to have a couple of fried eggs for breakfast; or you can make him look forward contentedly to his egg whites sunny-side up.

Whenever a Heart Wife is tense about her husband's meals, it invariably turns out to be because she assumes he will be on a life-long *diet.*

That word! Anyone who has ever been on a diet knows what it means: deprivation, hunger (especially for forbidden foods), willpower (or guilt), fussy, finicky meal preparation, temptation. A diet is hard; it is something you must constantly "watch." A diet is hell. And that is when it lasts only a week or two. Now it is going to be for a lifetime!

The wife thinks she must resign herself to endless preparation of two separate sets of meals—one for her husband, the other for the rest of the family.

Nonsense! Many husbands do go on a real, no-fooling diet for the same reason most people diet. To lose weight. But except for truly obese men, the largest part of weight loss is taken care of in the hospital. (Come to think of it, maybe *that* was the reason for your husband's hostility when he was in the hospital; anyone on a diet is apt to hate everyone in sight!) By the time most men are home—certainly after a few months—they no longer have to be on any kind of "diet," as that word is generally understood. They have to maintain their reduced weight and they have to keep their lowered cholesterol level where it is.

All that means is they should cut down on some things (beef, eggs, chocolate, etc.); they should eat some things in modified form (like nonfat or skimmed milk, polyunsaturated margarine); and their food should mostly be cooked in ways that may be different from those they are most accustomed to (broiled instead of fried, dry-grilled instead of basted, etc.). These are far from the rigors most people think of when they hear the word "diet."

It is true that some men also may go on a salt-restricted or low-sodium regimen, perhaps for quite a while. And for any heart patient who is also diabetic, there will be further restrictions in what he can eat and how his food is prepared.

But there is nothing in the goals of weight and cholesterol control that suggests or impels austerity, the slightest deprivation, unappetizing food, or tasteless food preparation. And that goes even for the somewhat sterner requirements of low-sodium or diabetic eating. The additional restrictions can make the job harder; but "harder" comes nowhere near meaning "impossible."

There is certainly nothing that suggests a need for separate meals! You never had the time to prepare separate meals before, did you? Well, do not start now! Not even special dishes. Again, it is a matter of attitude: you make it harder all around if you try to run a restaurant rather than a family dining table.

Instead, all you need do is plan tasty meals that everyone can eat, family-style—with everyone eating the same thing. (After all, the children deserve healthy food, too, don't they?)

What kind of family-style meals can you serve? Every kind! Styles of food preparation are technically known as "cuisines." French, Italian, Spanish, Chinese, etc. Most of us are already used to a mixture of the world's great cuisines. It will be fairly simple for you to master what amounts to just another: coronary cuisine—which has the advantage of shamelessly stealing appropriate dishes from every other cuisine in the world.

The important thing is your attitude, how you approach the whole subject of preparing food. If you go at it grimly, thinking of it as a diet, that is what it will be—for you, for your husband, for your whole family. If you simply make coronary cuisine your style of family food preparation, with meals every bit as tempting as they ever were (and a lot healthier!), it will simply become part of your family's eating habits.

Diets are hard, eating habits are easy. They are a reflection of one's natural inclinations.

After a remarkably short while, everyone in the family will be eating the right way, because that is simply what they are used to. One Heart Wife summed up the progression perfectly:

> It was hard at the start. I cooked two complete meals.
> But then I decided it wouldn't hurt the children, or me, to eat low-fat.
> At first I would add a little butter to theirs, whereas ours was

with margarine. But after a while there was no difference, so I stopped it. Finally, we were all eating the same things.

And the children got interested in how their father was eating. Now that they're young adults, they don't think of it as a problem—or even self-discipline. It's natural to them now.

In fact, they've gotten, well, intolerant. If they see their father eating the wrong things, they'll say, "Now you know you're just heading for another heart attack!"

To achieve results like that, you have to work at it. At first, but not for long. Once you have picked up the information you need and a few techniques, the whole process of planning meals, shopping, and cooking coronary cuisine will be second nature to you. Just as eating the right way will be second nature to your husband *and* to the rest of the family.

What You Have to Learn— and Where to Learn It

When we began research for this book, we were appalled to find out how much we did not know—and how much of what we "knew" was wrong. How should you get the information you need, and how can you be sure it is correct?

As always, the first step is *ask the doctor.*

But understand what information you should reasonably expect from him. He will give you the Grand Strategy: the goals of weight and cholesterol reduction and specifics on what your husband should eat and what he should avoid. For Tactics: the day-to-day details of what foods best accomplish the doctor's aims, where to get them, and how to make what you prepare delicious—for this information you obviously must look to other sources. The doctor's knowledge of casserole recipes is apt to be limited.

This all came up in a discussion with Annamarie Shaw, a registered nutritionist who is Program Associate in charge of

nutrition education and services for the Los Angeles County
Heart Association.

Mrs. Shaw put it this way:

> We always say to a wife who asks for a diet, "Ask your
> doctor—that is a medical question."
>
> But you may go to your doctor and ask a nutrition question.
> And very often he doesn't have nutrition information. Because
> the doctor would have to be a nutrition specialist, as well as a
> medical specialist.
>
> So we say, "Go to your doctor, he is the first line; he will set
> the limits, the prescription for the way your husband should eat.
> Then you may need help from a nutritionist to implement his
> prescription.
>
> "Call your Heart Association, or ask the doctor to refer you to
> somebody, or call the hospital dietician for specific information
> about food. This is *their* business. Just as he is a medical
> specialist, they are nutrition specialists."
>
> I cannot and will not prescribe. And no one else should
> prescribe a level of nutrition. No one!
>
> I get calls and they say, "My neighbor is on a such-and-such
> diet, and she tells me how great she feels. And I want a diet like
> she has for my husband." Or, "A man at a health food store told
> me about a diet . . ."
>
> I stop them right there. Your physician is the *only* one who
> can tell you.

Her statement was meant mostly for Heart Wives whose
husbands are on fairly routine weight- and cholesterol-level
maintenance programs. It has all the more force when applied to
husbands who need salt-restricted, low-sodium or diabetic
feeding. For those, working out basic menus in cooperation
with the doctor and a nutritionist is, if possible, even more
medically essential.

Mrs. Shaw went on to point out that how you get the basic,
prescriptive information you need is extremely important.
Everyone involved must be operating under the same Grand
Strategy, in all its details:

I learned this in family counseling. A man would have a heart attack or heart surgery and would be handed a diet sheet the day he left the hospital. He'd hand it to his wife—and she would just about have a heart attack when she saw it. I can't tell you how many people have told me this!

I often have a wife call me and say, "We're going home Friday. Will you give me a diet?" And I say, "Your doctor will undoubtedly give you a diet; check with the hospital dietician. Make sure you're there when the dietician gives your husband the instructions."

This must be a partnership!

If the wife tells the husband, "You can't have this because the doctor told me, or the dietician, or the chart says it," it often creates a lot of family tensions. The husband says, "Don't tell me what to do; the doctor didn't tell me that." Or, "I don't like that; you're just trying to change my life."

You know, this happens a lot.

So you must have a wedding, here, of the doctor, the dietician, the patient—*and* the family member who is going to be responsible for planning the menus, buying the food, and preparing the food.

The family "member," of course, is you. Now, what foods are all right? What foods are not? How can you tell? And how should you prepare them?

We mentioned some Heart Association pamphlets in Chapter Ten that are indispensable. They should be the first items in your own coronary-cuisine library. Here are the titles again:

— "Recipes for Fat-controlled, Low-cholesterol Meals"

— "The Way to a Man's Heart (A Fat-controlled, Low-cholesterol Meal Plan to Reduce the Risk of Heart Attack)"

— "Available Products for the Controlled-fat Diet"

— "Available Products for the Low-sodium Diet"

In addition, you will probably want some cookbooks. The three we will mention happen to be our favorites. You may find ones that suit you and your family better. Fine! One of the delights of coronary cuisine is the wide range of food and cooking styles it allows. Here are our own stand-bys:

The American Heart Association Cookbook (McKay, 1973)
(This is the bible for Heart Wives. It is authoritative and complete, with guidance for shopping, cooking, and serving meals, as well as an enormous number of recipes.)

Haute Cuisine for Your Heart's Delight (Potter, 1972) by Carol Cutler
(Subtitled, "A Low-Cholesterol Cook Book for Gourmets"; the accent is French, the recipes delicious!)

Cook to Your Heart's Content (Pacific Coast) by Dr. Daniel Liebowitz, Dr. W. Jann Brown, and Marlene Olness
(Subtitled, "On a Low-fat, Low-salt Diet," it is the best book we have come upon for meat-and-potatoes cookery—lean meat, and not too heavy on the potatoes, you understand!)

Now you are all set to go shopping.

Shopping: Can You Tell a Can by Its Label?

The only difference between shopping for coronary cuisine and however you shopped before is that now you must be a little more selective and brand-conscious. But once you have found out which foods are all right and which are not, shopping is a breeze.

How do you find out on your first trip, or when you see a new product? We will quote some authorities:

Mrs. Shaw: The best advice is, Read the label!

"Available Products": *Read the label.*
                                    In all cases read the labels. . . .
                                    Check labels.

Carol Cutler: . . . careful label reading is a must.

And just to make it official, this is from a Department of Health, Education and Welfare pamphlet describing the work of the Food and Drug Administration: "We urge you to read the label on all foods. . . ." Do you get a feeling that they are trying to tell you something? Right. And, taking the lesser with the greater, so are we: read the label!

The trouble is, as Mrs. Shaw also remarked, "Even when you read the label, you may not be too sure."

Don't panic. All she meant was that you must know what words to look for and what they mean when you find them. You should start out with a comprehensive list of foods, food products, and food ingredients that your husband should either cut out or cut down on. It must come from the doctor—or from a nutritionist or dietician who interprets the doctor's orders. Then you are ready to check labels.

Since 1938, manufacturers have been required to list all the ingredients in packages, cans, boxes, or bottles of processed food, and list them in order of quantity, starting with whatever the package contains most of, and working their way down. As you work your way down, you will run across some obscure ingredients in small type (a pocketbook-sized magnifying glass comes in handy). You may find your discovery unsettling. How can you tell whether an ingredient is all right for your husband or not if you have no idea what it is? We highly recommend a very handy paperback reference book called *A Consumer's Dictionary of Food Additives,* by Ruth Winter, (Crown, 1972) subtitled *Ingredients Harmful and Desirable Found in Packaged Foods with Complete Information for the Consumer,* it lists just about everything we have ever seen on a label and explains each with clarity.

That should take care of most of the label reading you must do. Except for the one word that causes Heart Wives more worry than any other: *fat.* But we are going to clear that up for you right now!

Living Off the Polyunsaturated Fat of the Land

Most of the confusion comes about over the difference between saturated and unsaturated (or polyunsaturated) fats. Cholesterol and monosaturated fats compound confusion. Roughly, here is the difference, in our own housewife terms, with an eye on result, not chemical accuracy:

SATURATED: Any kind of fat, from any source, that can increase the amount of cholesterol in the bloodstream when eaten in any form.
CHOLESTEROL: A particular kind of saturated fat. It is found only in living things (or something that comes from them—like eggs, milk, and milk products such as butter and cheese). It raises the cholesterol level in the bloodstream when eaten.
MONOSATURATED: A fat that neither raises nor lowers the amount of cholesterol in the bloodstream.
UNSATURATED: Any kind of fat that lowers the amount of cholesterol in the bloodstream. It is found only in vegetable fats.

Cholesterol is measured in milligrams. The other fats are measured in grams (there are 1,000 milligrams in a gram, just over 30 grams in an ounce). That is part of the confusion. For instance, shellfish used to be a star in coronary cuisine menus. Shrimp, crab, lobster, scallops, clams, and oysters are a tasty, low-calorie substitute for meat. They contain almost no fat. But then it was discovered that what fat they *do* contain is almost all cholesterol. To compare:

	Beef	Shrimp
Total fat per ounce	5–7 grams	less than ½ gram
Cholesterol per ounce	21 milligrams	38 milligrams

So shellfish are now featured less prominently in coronary cuisine.

When it comes to packaged foods, the problem is to interpret what you see on labels in terms of saturated or unsaturated fats. As of January 1, 1975, any food label that mentions fat content or cholesterol must give a complete analysis of how much of each kind is in that particular food.

Even so, you do well to *know* the most common sources for each kind of fat. We list only those sources with a significant amount of fat per ounce—with a couple of important notes.

Kinds of Foods	Saturated	Cholesterol	Monosaturated	Unsaturated
Meats	X	X		
Shellfish		X		
Fish	X *			
Poultry	X *			
Eggs		X		
Dairy Products	X	X		
Oils **				
coconut	X			
olive	X			
peanut			X	
corn ***				X
cottonseed				X
safflower				X
sesame seed				X
soybean				X
sunflower seed				X

* Almost all the fat is concentrated in the skin.
** You find them mostly in the form of margarines, cooking oils, and shortenings.
*** If a polyunsaturated oil has been treated to keep it fresh longer, it may become a saturated oil. The tip-off words to look for on the label are:
      hydrogenated
      hardened
      partially hardened or hydrogenated
      stabilized
      specially processed

When you look at the ingredients on a label, you can easily tell whether or not a margarine, shortening, cooking oil, or dressing contains an unacceptable amount of saturated fat by remembering this simple rule: The *first* oil listed must be specified as "liquid." After that, if some partially hardened oil is listed, it will not matter. But if the first oil listed is *anything* but liquid (or, of course, coconut oil in any form), do not buy that product. A Heart Association pamphlet gives this example:

Brand A is acceptable:	*Brand X is NOT acceptable:*
liquid safflower oil	partially hydrogenated corn oil
partially hardened	liquid corn oil
soybean oil	nonfat milk, etc.
nonfat dry milk, etc.	

Remember, we are talking about the official, legally required list of ingredients. The advertising blurbs you may also see on a label do not necessarily mean much. The manufacturer is not allowed to lie, but he is allowed to be highly selective about what truth he tells. The blurb can be pretty misleading. For instance, Mrs. Shaw pointed this out about the word "pure":

When a label says "pure vegetable fat"—doesn't that sound marvelous!

Or you see a big, beautiful bottle of vegetable oil, and it says on the label, "High in Polyunsaturates"—but down here, first on the list of ingredients, in tiny print, it says "Specially Processed Vegetable Oil."

So you buy it—and perhaps pay a few pennies extra because it's high in unsaturates, but you don't know that the "specially processed" means hydrogenated, to preserve shelf life.

If the label tells you just "Vegetable Oil" and doesn't tell you what kind, be suspicious.

We would be more than suspicious; we would be off, in search of another product whose manufacturer was either more considerate or less sneaky.

The same goes for any "imitation" products. As Mrs. Shaw put it:

> I'm suspicious of "imitation" *anything*. It is generally made with coconut oil—because coconut oil tastes better, lasts longer, and costs the maker less.

They could have fooled us. Fact is, they did for a long time! After all, imitation diamonds are one thing. But what is there in sour cream that would make it necessary to imitate the original? The cream, obviously. And, sure enough, all imitation sour cream containers we have seen proudly proclaim their status as "nondairy" products. This sounds good, right? But look at the ingredient list: "coconut oil" leads all the rest. You might just as well have had the genuine article, both in point of calories and saturated fat. (And, incidently, price.) There is somewhat more excuse for "nondairy" coffee creamers. At least they do not require refrigeration. But every one we have seen is made with—you guessed it, anonymous "vegetable fat."

It is not hard to read labels—when you know what words to look for and what they mean when you find them.

Bringing It All Together

Once you have found out which products contain saturated fats and which do not, you have one more thing to remember: *In terms of calories, fat is fat.*

In the fight against high blood cholesterol, the polyunsaturated fats are the "good guys," the saturated fats are the "blue meanies" and the monosaturates are by-standers who do not want to get involved. But they *all* have exactly the same number of calories: nine per gram.

So you cannot load up your menu with fats. Not even the good guys. Because the *twin* goals of coronary cuisine are keeping weight down (which means total calories) and keeping cholesterol down (which means total saturated fat and total cholesterol eaten).

The totals give you a lot of maneuvering room.

For instance, all meat contains saturated fat. But veal contains less than beef, chicken contains less than duck. And fish contains least of all. Except for shellfish. You see how the balance works.

The rest of coronary cuisine is no harder than shopping. Just as you no longer pick up any old thing at the market, you no longer prepare it any old way. But the rules are few and simple, and the result is gratifying: weight reduction is easier and lowered cholesterol is assured. And the taste can be superb!

As Miss Cutler's book shows, almost any recipe can be juggled, maneuvered, defatted, and decaloried with no loss to taste. In her Introduction, Miss Cutler writes:

> I don't want to boast, but I have made every dish in this book with good results. They have been served to knowledgeable members of the family, friends, and even finicky French gourmets. The last mentioned, if they had known they were eating low-cholesterol meals, would have found fault with the preparation. They did not know, and they didn't complain. In fact, many of them praised the lightness of the cuisine.

You do not have the same advantage of surprise, but you do not need it. Substitutions for most recipes simply do not affect the dish's original taste. We defy anyone to detect a difference between French toast or meat loaf made with two egg whites and the same made with a whole egg. The only difference is in cholesterol, but that is all the difference in the world for coronary cuisine. And for your husband's health.

Coronary Cuisine Cookery—
What You Do with What You've Got

You are already an experienced coronary-cuisine cook. You just did not know it. But there is nothing in the basics that is new or strange. It is simply a matter of knowing which of your cooking skills should be used. After you have added a few new twists of your own, you will be an *expert* coronary-cuisine cook. As one Heart Wife said:

It's been fun!
I have a lot of fun cooking this way—disguising things, changing things, fooling them all! It's been *fun!* And it really isn't difficult, you know. You take your scissors and take the skin off the chicken and the fat off the meat; you learn to make gravies and skim the fat. You argue with the butcher—you say, "No, I want it trimmed"; you insist on it, and after a while they listen to you.
Really, I've had a ball!

Of course, she enjoyed cooking *before* her husband's heart attack. Coronary cuisine will not make you enjoy cooking any more than you did, if you didn't. But it certainly will make your husband lovingly delighted at how good are what he feared would be dreary meals!

Here are some basic rules and techniques. We quote them directly from the Heart Association pamphlets' recipes—with a few comments of our own.

Meats
Even lean meat has fat in it. Here are some ways to reduce the saturated fat in meat:

Use a rack to drain off the fat when broiling, roasting, or baking. Instead of basting with drippings, keep meat moist by pouring wine, tomato juice, or bouillon over it.

Cook a day ahead of time: stew, boiled meat, soup stock, or other dishes in which fat cooks into the liquid. After the food has been refrigerated, the hardened fat can be removed from the top.

Make gravies after the fat has hardened and can be removed from the liquid.

Broil, rather than pan-fry, meats such as hamburger, lamb chops, pork chops, and steak.

When a recipe calls for browning the meat first, try browning it under the broiler instead of in a pan.

If you do not already have a pan with a removable rack, it is an excellent investment; alternatively, you can buy packages of foil broiling pans with built-in serrated bottoms that easily serve the same purpose.

The technique given for broiling instead of pan-frying is fine, but the illustration of meats may be misleading. Even broiled, the meats mentioned are pretty rich in cholesterol and are subject to whatever your doctor has told you about how much meat to serve.

Vegetables

Vegetables can be made more tempting by adding herbs and spices. For example, these combinations add new and subtle flavors: rosemary with peas, cauliflower, and squash; oregano with zucchini; dill with green beans; marjoram with brussels sprouts, carrots, and spinach; basil with tomatoes.

Start with a small quantity (one-eighth to one-half teaspoon to a package of frozen vegetables); then let your own and your family's taste be your guide.

Chopped parsley and chives, sprinkled on just before serving, also enhance the flavor of many vegetables.

Try cooking vegetables in vegetable oil, adding a little water during cooking if needed. Use one to two teaspoons of oil for each serving, place in a skillet with tight cover, season, and cook over very low heat until vegetables are done.

Vegetable oil is good, but for perking up the flavor of vegetables, the best method we have run across is to cook them in chicken or beef stock. That adds little in calories, lots in flavor, and can be creatively combined with herbs.

Incidently, the reason they may need perking up, which is not spelled out in these instructions, is the habit most of us get into of dousing vegetables with butter and salt before serving, or cooking them up with fatty meats, such as bacon or salt pork. The reason is flavor—and the result is coronary holocaust. Vegetables are among the few low-calorie foods you were used to serving. But when swimming in butter or bacon grease, they are almost as fattening as anything this side of strawberry shortcake. Using margarine is not better, not even polyunsat-urate. Fat is fat, remember?

Using Vegetable Oils

The liquid vegetable oils or margarines high in polyunsat-urates can be used in many ways in cooking that requires the use of fat. For example:

To brown lean meats, and to pan- or oven-fry fish and poultry;

To sauté onions and other vegetables for soup;

In cream sauces and soups made with skimmed milk;

In whipped or scalloped potatoes with skimmed milk added;

For making hot breads, pie crust, and cakes;

For popping corn, and making cocktail snacks;

In casseroles made with dried peas or beans;

In browning rice and for Spanish rice or curried rice;

In cooking dehydrated potatoes and other prepared foods that call for fat to be added;

For pancakes or waffles.

As with meat, you must not take the listing of foods as permission to use them very liberally. It is important to keep in mind the stated purpose of any recipe book. This particular pamphlet is dedicated to low fat; it mentions foods as examples of use, not recommendations for your shopping list.

That is not *all* there is to coronary-cuisine cookery. But it is essentially all you have to know to get well on your way to expert status.

As a bonus, here is what Miss Cutler points out as some side benefits of shopping and cooking for coronary cuisine:

... it is an economical way of eating, since vegetables, fish, and poultry are used much more and are among the less expensive items that go into the shopping basket.... What meats are bought are not prime cuts, well marbled with fat, but leaner, cheaper cuts. Dinner parties become easier to give, since much cooking is done in advance. Why? To save time for the hostess and so that food can be chilled in order to skim off all fat. There is still another bonus: many classic dishes, like Coq au Vin, taste better reheated.

Eating Out

In reality, eating out is more of a problem than eating home. There are more temptations in a restaurant, and there is no choice when you are at someone else's home, where it may be roast beef or nothing. And, either place, you cannot be sure about ingredients or methods or preparation.

The only way around both problems (except to always stay home, which may not be possible and is surely no fun) depends on knowledge and attitude.

In restaurants it means knowing which are *probably* acceptable foods, *probably* cooked in acceptable ways. The Heart Association offers a guide to eating out. The degree of their own confidence in it is reflected in its format. Unlike their other pamphlets, which are well-produced, multipaged, sometimes illustrated in color, "Eating Out on the Fat-controlled Diet" is a page-and-a-half mimeographed sheet. The Heart Association is not particularly happy with it. The trouble is, there cannot be a truly authoritative guide to the problem, since nearly everything depends on the cooperation of the restaurant or host. If, as "Eating Out" suggests, you, "SPECIFY NO GRAVY, BUTTER, OR REGULAR MARGARINE TO BE USED," you can only hope someone is listening.

But with knowledge, you can select foods that give you a better chance of avoiding excessive fats and excessive calories.

At a friend's house or at a set-menu banquet it is certainly permissible to explain your problem. Friends will probably be quite willing to adjust their menus or their methods or both when they understand. If not—well, are you sure they are "friends"? And if no one on the banquet committee will help, remember that doggie bags can carry meals in two directions. *That* will show them!

Your final line of defense is attitude. Miss Cutler expressed that attitude almost perfectly:

> In the modern world, 100 percent control of your diet is difficult. When traveling, dining with friends, and eating in restaurants, it is hard to avoid high-cholesterol food. What I propose is that you maintain strict control over what you eat at home every day. Then, on the occasion when a quivering soufflé is placed before you—enjoy it. But the soufflé must be the exception, not the rule. By following a careful diet most of the time, you have, so to speak, cholesterol credit in the bank. So you can cash in that credit when you dine out from time to time.

Our only quarrel with that is her image of "cholesterol credit in the bank." In fairness, Miss Cutler's valuable book is meant for everyone, not just those with an already demonstrated cardiac condition. But the most useful attitude for you and your husband to develop is not one that sees excess of any fat (Miss Cutler uses "cholesterol" as a shorthand term for all fat) as a positive treat, or any sort of a reward. It is *not* like building up "cholesterol credit," which you may then feel free to "cash in" from time to time. Using the same analogy, it is more like meeting payments at the bank, not making deposits. Even if you overpay one week, you are not *entitled* to underpay the next.

You do build up a "cholesterol credit," but it is a long-range credit, not one to be squandered at the first opportunity, any more than an alcoholic who has gone ten years without a drink would toast his victory in champagne.

With the right sort of long-range attitude, and with an ever-growing awareness of how to plan, shop, and cook, plus how to pick and choose among already prepared dishes when you eat out, there is nothing to be nervous about.

A Short After-Dinner Speech

Some men are easy to cook for, others are difficult, with or without the complication of myocardial infarctions. That is not going to change. But, then, neither will the degree of care, attention, and work that you must put into pleasing your husband's tastes. The man who was pleased with the meals you served before can be just as pleased with the meals you serve now. As for the modifications necessary in what he eats, and how they are made—well, he knows (and has a considerable stake in not forgetting) the reason and need for a change.

Your attitude will have a lot to do with it. How will he adjust to "a heart-patient's diet," if that is what you serve? Grudgingly, uncomfortably, and worst of all, perhaps temporarily. In short, pretty much the same way anyone takes to any diet.

How will your husband and your family—and you—adjust to coronary cuisine? You will eat it right up!

As we said at the start, it all depends on you.

CHAPTER
20

How to Be a Shrew—
With Delicate Grace and
Charm

We mean the title of this chapter literally, just as it stands, for all the seeming self-contradiction implicit in the notion of ferocious charm. Call it the iron hand in the velvet glove. Call it the paradox of feminine resolve. Or just call it being a Heart Wife.

For, make no mistake, there will come times all throughout your life as a Heart Wife when you will have to be absolutely ruthless, totally remorseless, devoid of the least softness or consideration for others. No matter how you used to be or how little you relish your stern duty.

Mrs. R illustrated the point and the need for strategic shrewishness with a story she told us. When her husband was released from the CCU, he was moved into a semiprivate room, the only one available, she was told. The room was fine, the other patient was not. He was a very old man, querulous, sure he was dying, and determined to share the news with the world:

> He did nothing but grump and groan all night long, ... "Ah! I'm dying, I'm dying!"
> And during the day, the wife would come in and scream.

Mr. R had had a massive coronary, with some complications that had brought him close to death himself. But he had not died. He had recovered, though it took better than two weeks in the CCU before the doctor was willing even to quote odds on his chances. Now here he was, his rest and even sleep disturbed. True, the roommate may well have been right to be bitter in his complaint against the universe. And, right or wrong, he unarguably had a "right" to say what he thought the way he wanted to. But he had no right to endanger Mrs. R's husband.

Not to her way of thinking, at least.

Would it be to yours, if your husband were involved? Silly question! You would surely object to any atmosphere for your husband's recovery that included the sight and sound of a self-proclaimed dying man who insists on making his proclamation long and loud.

But wait! Objecting is one thing, correcting quite another. After all, the poor, dying old man will be so horribly embarrassed if your objection amounts to much more than inner seething. Your husband may be embarrassed too. Anyway, what can be done? And by whom? Those visibly overworked nurses and staff members? The doctor who looks as though he would settle for a spell in any bed, under any conditions? It is not as though any of them are deliberately making things tough for you and your husband; everyone has been sweetness and light. And they are not lying to you about things, either. You can see for yourself that there really is not another bed available in a room anywhere on the floor. Besides, the doctor knows; if he does not see fit to worry, what right have you to make any fuss? Who are you to demand? Do you want to be known as a troublemaker?

Of course not. So what do you do?

You raise bloody hell until they find another room, or arrange another room, or build another room, for all you care! They can look on another floor for a room, or transfer some poor soul who is either unconscious, himself dying, or so well and chipper he will not mind the querulous old man. How they do it does not matter. You will see to it, though, that they *do* do it!

That's what you do.

Sweetly, if that helps—or does not hinder; but forcefully, tenaciously, and in a way no one will mistake as being anything other than implacable.

Let Mrs. R put it completely in perspective:

I found out, as a wife, that you're not going to get your husband changed to another room unless you holler a little bit and *you* see that he's changed.

If I didn't get him changed, nobody else was going to.

But we just agreed that you did not want to be known as a troublemaker, didn't we? Sure. Who does? But how do you feel about being known as a widow? Okay, we are playing a game with the phrase "known as," but it is much to the point. One is a matter of reputation, the other is a matter of chilling fact. You know you are not a natural-born troublemaker, one who takes some bizarre delight in unreasonable demands. So if what you must do on some occasions causes you to become known as one, it does not materially affect what you actually are. On the other hand, if you do nothing about a situation of such disturbing magnitude that it contributes to your husband's death—and you have done nothing because doing something might create the false impression that you actually like throwing your weight around—you will not just be "known" as a widow, you will be one. Incontrovertibly, and not by mistaken reputation.

Besides, how people feel about you or think of you is not the point. Not now. Your husband's recovery is the only point; and when you run into situations where someone is trying to make that point the hard way, you must act. Just like a shrew. Just like a Heart Wife. At those moments the words should be interchangeable. You must be a shrew who cares only about her husband's well-being. Not people's feelings, not the doctor's opinion or exhaustion, not the nurse's harassment, not the old man's plight or his wife's natural perturbation. Only your husband's recovery.

Is every annoyance really all that serious? Every one a matter of his recovering or not?

Who knows? Probably not, but you surely dare not take a chance. Whenever there is a situation you feel is detrimental to your husband's present health and future recovery, it would be folly to stand aside on the vague hope that, well, maybe it will not really have all that bad an effect on him. Because, if it does, it could be a lot worse than bad; it could be horrible. At the same time, the worst effect your action could have is mere unpleasantness. And you will get over the unpleasantness of having to be unpleasant a good deal more easily and quickly than you will get over the complications of a slow recovery, or the nonrecovery, of your husband.

It is the difference between hazarding health and hazarding "feelings." People get over hurt feelings; no one gets over dying.

And even from the viewpoint of your personal survival as a woman and wife who feels reasonably good about herself, it makes no sense to risk the feelings of guilt you will inevitably have about your husband if you are not morally certain you have done everything you can to help him. Especially when all you truly risk is "popularity" with people who either are strangers or who, if close to you, should know better.

Do you remember the Heart Wife who said she just did not "have time to indulge the trivialities of my friends"? A different Heart Wife spoke to the same general point in a way that is both more forceful and more pertinent to your entire situation in dealing with the world, friends or not:

> My mission was to get him well—and the hell with everybody else's feelings. . . .

That is not to say you should go out of your way to be abrasive. Or that you will often have to. Under the circumstances, you can expect most people you come in contact with, or who come in contact with your husband, to be considerate and to want to do what they can to help. Not just when he is in the hospital, not just when he is recuperating at home, but for the rest of your lives as a cardiac couple. But people have an un-canny knack of being—*human.* They make mistakes, they forget to remember, they become overwhelmed with their own problems and lose sight of other people's problems. Within limits, that is perfectly all right. As the years pass for you, the level of annoyance from other people that you can tolerate for your husband keeps going up. But it will never reach whatever the high mark was before the attack. Or it shouldn't, anyway.

But perhaps you never thought of there being a limit before. There was, however, as you will readily see at a moment's reflection. There always were certain people and certain annoyances that you instinctively knew were bad for your husband long before it became a matter of health. You shielded him (as, very likely, he shielded you from certain people, places, and things that infallibly drive you up the wall). The heart attack does not change the principle of what you must do, just the threshold of action.

So the "being a shrew" part of this process is perfectly clear. The delicate grace and charm is not. Yet. Maybe even the need for it is a little murky. Okay you say, you see the need to adopt or develop a tough-mindedness that may always have been alien to your nature; you see the necessity of speaking in ways and doing things that would have horrified you before your husband's heart attack. But if you are going to do it, why not . . . *do* it? Why the qualifications? For most people it is hard enough to be a thorough-going, effective shrew at all, in hot blood and under full steam. Start with the nice distinctions and who knows if you will be able to carry through? Anyhow, why bother?

Britain's ex-Prime Minister Winston Churchill once wrote that, "When you have to kill a man, it costs nothing to be polite." He might have added that, in fact, it can cost you something very dear indeed to be anything but polite. It costs your objectivity, humanity, and sense of proportion. The more distasteful the task, the more important it is that you undertake it on pure principle, being sure that you do frightful things only under the prod of necessity, never because you are developing a taste for being frightful.

Just because, over the years to come, there will be those times when you must be a shrew, it is not at all the same as saying that you must become one. Indeed, if you do become one, it will defeat the very purpose of being one. Your changed personality will begin to taint relations with your husband, making his recovery and adjustment harder than if you had never bothered to interpose yourself between him and what you saw as dangerous people and experiences. After all, no one has the power to upset him that you do; and no one wants to live with a shrew.

How can you be one without becoming one?

The most effective way is to lower the amount of shrewish- ness necessary. That means interposing your personality be- fore a situation becomes a storm. It is also the kindest way, since it lets you accomplish your goal with delicate grace and charm, rather than naked, unabashed shrewishness.

You can generally see the storm clouds on the horizon: you *know* certain people in certain situations upset your husband. And they are often people or situations he takes in stride, even happily, when he is feeling all right. They are often family, close friends, or business associates—in general, people toward whom he feels bonds of love or familiarity or obligation so strong that they resist even the knife of basic incompatibility. Usually, only people close to a man have the power to upset him to a degree that makes it imperative for you to step in ahead of time if you are to avoid trouble. In a way, that is fortunate. Because it is only such people that you can do much about beforehand. The casual annoyer brings his mischief to your husband with no warning: the irritating waiter, the infuriating salesclerk, the aggressively offensive guest at someone else's party. These cannot be anticipated. But, then, their power to churn your husband is limited enough so that you can deal with them at the time. Aunt Hattie, Uncle Boris, and your husband's no-good nephew are another matter. They can induce apoplexy within seconds, if given an opportunity to get started.

The same goes for situations as for people. The familiar

situations are the most dangerous but are also the easiest to deal
with. For one thing, situations do not surprise you. An individual you may be eyeing warily can suddenly behave like a
living jewel (and vice versa, of course). But a situation you
identify as essentially rotten is not likely to improve.

One Heart Wife realized that, weighed the probable effect
on her husband of a situation she saw looming, and took the
necessary steps—first of which was telling her husband what she
was going to do, since the situation she saw needing correction
was one that involved a necessary modification in her husband's
former gregarious hospitality. Her analysis and her actions
make up, in effect, a perfect case history and example of the
necessary technique:

> I said, "Honey, I've thought so much about this since you've
> been here in the hospital, this running a 'hotel' that we do."
> I mean, it's like a boarding house, that's what our home was.
> We both wanted it like that—people dropping in, coming to stay
> for visits. But now?
> I said, "We can't have it anymore. I'm tired, I'm getting
> exhausted—and it isn't going to be good for you. I don't want to
> hurt anyone's feelings, but I know I'm going to have to stop it."

You'll have to, too. There will be situations in which you will
simply have to step in and lay waste to whomever or whatever is
threatening, or might threaten, your husband's recovery.

Now cutting a man off from his friends must be reckoned the
actions of a considerable shrew. But there is nothing in what the
Heart Wife said to her husband, nothing in the explanation she
told us she gave to the people who had gotten used to feeling the
couple was holding perpetual open house, nothing that is in the
slightest shrewish. Nothing. Because it is not a case of raving or
ranting, of throwing the rascals out, it is the calm statement of
what must be done, with firm assurance that she could and
would do what she had to do. It cost her nothing to be
polite—and might have cost quite a bit to be otherwise.

You indeed may have to do some hollering from time to time.
But it is not necessary to assume that you will. The hollering

comes when you are quite sure, either because you have already tried or because you are morally certain ahead of time, that the tranquillity you want for your husband will be impossible to achieve without hollering. The hollering itself is certainly not what you want. In addition to the deleterious effect on you (being a shrew can get to be a habit, like anything else—one that is eventually worse for your health than smoking and worse for your attractiveness than nail-biting), starting off at a holler can undermine your program of controlled shrewishness. The problem is most acute for people who have always been rather retiring and unassertive. Hollering can be for that sort of Heart Wife what alcohol is for a naturally timid man who contemplates a fistfight. It is Dutch courage, nothing more, and rather than prime yourself or stimulate yourself for what you must do, you should train yourself to do it, not in a temper and not with the crutch of self-induced righteous anger, but coolly and efficiently—ruthlessly, if you will—because it must be done and you realize the need for doing it.

The need for cultivating a talent for the sort of shrewishness we mean is most evident when it comes to dealing with people who are essentially close friends and with potentially troublesome members of your immediate family. And if the charm does not do it—well, the overriding consideration is to achieve the necessary results. That comes first, and you must always be prepared to go as far as need be with the sheer shrewishness part of the formula. That is exactly why you would take the trouble to try delicate grace and charm first: you presumably do not want to hurt, discomfort, or alienate people who have been close to your husband.

Take friends who visit, for example. We have already discussed various techniques for handling visitors in Chapters Six and Twelve, and this is not a review. But as we skim over some details, notice how they apply *in general* to the whole range of problems that may call for some shrewishness on your part.

First you talk to potential visitors ahead of time, all grace and charm, with the assumption that they are as anxious to do what is best for your husband as you are. Perhaps you arrange a signal to let them know visiting hours are over. There is nothing shrewish about that. You preserve your husband's rest, without creating unpleasant tension between him and a close friend or relative who feels that close affection somehow renders longer visits unharmful.

Contrast that technique of charm to a flat-out demand that visitors leave after so many minutes. The latter is shrewishness. But . . . so is the first! With the saving addition of delicate grace and charm.

The same distinction can apply even to people who, for any reason other than malevolence (those you can do without altogether!), cannot bring themselves to cooperate. Sure, you could straight-out tell such people that they are not allowed in your house until such-and-such a date. Period, end of sentence. And, very possibly, end of a friendship that in sunnier times may be of value and importance to your husband. That would be a shame.

You can likely achieve the same result of keeping certain people away from your husband for however many weeks you think necessary, with at worst only moderately bruised feelings. You might start out by blaming the doctor. (It is only fair to tell him what you are doing and why.) He has forbidden visitors, but, naturally, the people in question will be the *very first* to be notified the absolute second the doctor lifts his silly ban.

It does not matter much whether it is believed or not. Remember that you are dealing with someone on whom you are perfectly prepared to exercise pure shrewishness; this, instead, is quintessential shrewishness with delicate-grace-and-charm. You give the person an out, except that this out is one, final attempt to find an alternative to "Get lost," without risking any misunderstanding as to the basic message of "don't call us, we'll call you."

Just do not forget that behind the sweetness and light must always be a steely, uncompromising determination that you *will,* damn it, achieve the result you want, and by shrewishness—undiluted, unadulterated, and unashamed—if need be. All we are saying is, why start with the ultimate weapon? Why risk "overkill" of affections? Why crush walnuts with a steam hammer—at least before you have given that cute Hansel and Gretel nutcracker a try?

There is another reason, beyond preserving friendships. With some people and some situations the time will come when the kissing does have to stop, when even escalated "charm" gets you nowhere. You will be better able to judge when that time has come if you have been practicing the art of gauging the effectiveness of appropriately heightened shrewishness, with reciprocally diminished grace and charm. And you will keep your eventual shrewishness that much more credible for not having overexposed it. If you become known as one who is always being shrewish about the slightest infraction of what you establish as rules for behavior around your husband, those from whom you want to protect him will build immunity even to whatever final degrees of shrillness you can attain. By taking the measured approach we have been discussing, you train both yourself and others to appreciate all the more those moments when even the densest pest must say, "Hey! She really means it; she's . . . mad!" You will also be a more accurate judge of when those moments have arrived.

It comes down to a clear, unambiguous realization of what you owe to whom, of what, finally, is important.

It is completely up to you, of course. But we can assume that, like most Heart Wives, you put your husband's welfare first. Now that sounds so automatic as to seem like a simpleminded platitude. But it is not, because you will continually be called upon to balance probable or possible damage to your husband's health against almost certain damage to other people's feelings or sensibilities. Sometimes it will involve an entire network of other people's feelings. And, as we have already suggested, the balance changes as the years pass. That is, feelings are always much less important than life, but the probability of jeopardy to one or the other changes. No matter. Once you are clear as to what comes first with you, it is much easier to make the sensible decision, now or ten years from now, even if it remains a hard, unpleasant one.

Mrs. G is one of the most charming, attractive, and totally gentle people we have ever met. But there was a problem: her husband's doctor was not really a cardiologist. In this case, Mrs. G considered the doctor in question to be really a *non*cardiologist, and that he was on the case for reasons other than his competence as a doctor. Right or wrong, Mrs. G felt that he was wrong for her husband. She told us:

> When my father-in-law had a heart attack, we stuck to one doctor, and I kept saying it was a mistake.
>
> My husband has a typical male trait: for example, I changed milkmen the other day, to Brand X, because it's a purer product, and my husband said, "How can you tell that man you're letting him go *after all these years!*" And I said, "Because I think our family comes first—and I think Brand X is a purer product and I'm going to get it."
>
> It took me a long time to come to that point of view.
>
> With my father-in-law, I kept saying, "Why don't we have somebody else come in—you know, another opinion?" But they both said, "It's an insult to this doctor." He is also a social friend, which I think is a mistake for that very reason. They said, "Having someone else would be insulting; you're questioning his ability!"
>
> But *this* time, when it was *my* husband and I gave it some thought, I just didn't care anymore. I didn't care! I told him, "I'm calling in someone in addition to be on the case."

We say it again: "right or wrong." Mrs. G had substantial reasons for feeling that there should be another doctor on the case. When situations come up for you, it will not matter one bit that you may seem to be dealing in areas where you have no pretense to expertise, opposing your judgment against those who are expert. The fact is, you are not on such alien ground as it might appear.

The distinction between Mrs. G's decision in two seemingly

identical instances of a single problem is revealing. When it was a question of her father-in-law, she had no final responsibility and no right to go further than a reasonably emphatic statement of her opinion. If her father-in-law and her husband felt that, no, the old friend's feelings were more important than his medical skill (or, of course, if they felt she was wrong about that skill), it was not up to her to insist. So she did not. When her husband's life was at stake, it became another matter. There, she did have not only the right but the duty to insist that her opinion prevail. Nobody else's opinion mattered, except as she might consult other opinions to help shape her own. The subject, in both cases, was *not* medicine; it was the best interest of a particular person.

Your husband, your family, yourself. They come ahead of even self-doubt. Another Heart Wife whose husband's heart attack was very mild and occurred nearly twenty-five years ago, before the age of modern diagnostic techniques, told us that her husband had been sent home from the hospital after two days, and his heart attack was not diagnosed until three weeks later. We asked what, in retrospect, she thinks she would have done differently:

> When I thought he didn't seem "right" and I wanted them to keep him in the hospital, they said, No—he's all right at home. So I thought, "Well, so I'm wrong."
>
> I should have insisted.
>
> Today I would. I don't mind telling off doctors. Lately none of us does.

By "us," she meant Heart Wives. Including, hopefully, you. But who are you to tell doctors their business? What gives you the right? Easy. You are the one person involved who cares more about your husband's welfare than about any other aspect of the situation. Doctors have their own families, their own concerns, egos, hang-ups; and they have other patients with claims on their time, attention, and energies as valid as your husband's. You have only one "patient," only one interest.

In addition, you are far and away the closest, most knowledgeable observer and student of your husband's condition, the one person involved who is most likely to be able to just *know* that something is wrong, no matter what the lab report says. And you are the one who loses the most if, indeed, it is the doctor, not you who is mistaken. That alone gives you paramount right.

None of which is to say we think your *medical* judgment is comparable to that of the doctors. It is your personal judgment we are backing; and we would back that of any wife about her husband against any doctor. Because, save for hysterics, a wife who feels so strongly that something is wrong, even in the face of competent medical opinion and assurances, and in the absence of some reasonable explanation from the doctor to account for the difference in opinion—that wife must have a point. And she certainly has a duty to defend her case in the face of any opposition. If you are in such a position, it is up to you to be totally intransigent. Maybe your husband's "eyes look tired" or his "color looks wrong." If any of the private little telltales that are, for you, absolute indicators of his health say "danger," tell the doctor. An answer such as, "Well, yes, he is supposed to seem tired after walking two miles; I want that and expect that," is perfectly suitable. That is a medical decision the doctor is much better able to make than you are. On the other hand, your wariness should be triggered by any answer that does not account for your considered opinion as to the state of your husband's health, but seems instead to dismiss it as faulty observation. "He is supposed to look that way" is acceptable; "You are wrong about how he looks or what it means" is not.

We used the example of doctors because the decision to exercise shrewishness is commonly the most difficult when dealing with them. You tremble at the thought of you, an amateur, encroaching on their professional field. Our point is that, quite the contrary, they are amateurs in the "field" of knowing and observing your husband, while you are that art-and-science's foremost practitioner. It is a vital point, because it is the same in many other instances, with lesser authorities in

less learned fields. Or with outstanding authorities in trivial
fields. Because the field of their expertise is irrelevant.
Remember Mrs. R. The old man in the next bed had a wife, too.
And that wife may have been dismayed over the effect on her
own husband of the criticism of his behavior implicit in Mrs. R's
insistence on a transfer. Would there be a bad effect on the old
man? If his wife said so. She alone can be counted the expert in
that field. Had she concluded that the effect would be awful and
had she said as much to Mrs. R, we would back her judgment
against any doctor or any nurse who pooh-poohed the notion
and tried to assure her that, no, her husband wasn't really going
to mind having his roommate moved to another room. But from
Mrs. R's viewpoint, the effect on the old man is irrelevant. She
does not dispute the opinion of the other wife and she can
certainly try her best to mitigate any ill effect on the old man.
But that is the grace and delicate charm part. The result is the
only thing of the moment: her husband is going to get out of that
atmosphere. Out! How and with what spirit is negotiable.
Whether he does, or how soon, is not. He is—and immediately;
and that's that.

Part of your job, remember, is taking into account those
forces that might now disturb your husband which would not
have disturbed him, or called for any action from you, before.
One Heart Wife found herself having to chase little children
from their play because her husband could not rest due to their
noise. Another Heart Wife found herself using vocabulary and
tone most appropriate to Marine Corps boot camps when
talking to the phone company about installation of a necessary
extension. Neither liked doing it, neither fancied herself for
what she did. Both just did it. Effectively. Because first things
come first—and with your husband's recovery in even possible
balance, little children at their play or the self-respect of de-
fenseless utilities employees just don't count too much. They
will, again; as your husband gets better, as the years roll on, first
things will still be first, but by a narrowing margin. As long as
you keep in mind that they are first, by however slight a margin,
you cannot go far wrong.

What kind of woman would forbid little children their charming, innocent games? The kind of woman who has a husband who must rest and is being constantly disturbed by shouting outside his window. What kind of woman would dare drag doctor, exhausted from long hours saving people's lives, out of bed in the middle of the night? And then call in another doctor if not satisfied that the one is not taking the case seriously? The kind of woman whose husband has a heart condition and is experiencing inexplicable pains. The kind of woman whose "mission is to get him well."

If you can do it with delicate grace and charm, all the better. If you have to say "To hell with everybody's feelings," so be it.

If the choice is between being the sweetest, best-liked *widow* in the whole town and being the best-loved wife and mother in one single family, we know which we would choose. Make your choice, if it comes to that; and make up your mind that you will do whatever is necessary to make it stick.

CHAPTER

21

Heartfelt Thanks

Now don't get us wrong. We are not suddenly going ga-ga and misty-eyed over the delights of coronary occlusions. We are not going to treat you to musings on how lucky you are that, oh, goodie, your husband had a heart attack.

Earlier a Heart Wife said that if it takes a heart attack to bring people to their senses about how they are living and how they should be living, then, so be it—and we admitted that she had a point there, since the alternative is quite often unhappy lives and failed marriages. But the flaw in such thinking is the fact that it is not really a matter of alternatives for you and your husband. There is no question but that your life, your husband's life, your life together can be better after the heart attack than before. No question at all. But it will not be because of the heart attack. It will be because of what the two of you do. You will have yourselves to thank, not the heart attack.

This is no mere quibble over words.

It is probably still too soon for you to *feel* what we are about to say. You may have to take it on faith. The ultimate problem does not become particularly acute for several years after the heart attack, certainly not until all the novelty of being a cardiac couple wears off. But if you can accept what we are going to point out on the basis of our own experiences and that of just about all the other Heart Wives we know, you will keep yourself, and help keep your husband, out of the way of some serious attitude problems in the future, ones that can impede your smooth, long-time adjustment.

There are two opposite ways of looking at your husband's heart attack that are equally possible, equally dangerous, and equally wrong. Both are paralyzing. Both help throw up a psychological block to doing what you must do in the long run.

The first is the "Silver Lining" approach. The other is the "Worm in the Bud" approach. The common peril they share is the fact that both are perfectly natural and logical extensions of accurate, supportive, and essential ways of thinking about your life and about the consequences of the heart attack.

What makes them all the worse is that they can so easily alternate; and what makes "all the worse" absolutely awful is that once you find yourself swinging to one attitude, the only corrective measure possible is a conscious, sharp mental pull in the opposite direction. So you stagger along on an emotional tightrope, teetering farther and farther off balance, first to one side, then to the other—always off balance.

The "Silver Lining" fallacy is to con yourself and your husband into believing that the heart attack was all for the best. There you were, living lives of quiet (or noisy) desperation, when, ah! came the warning. Weren't you lucky! Because that is what it took. And now you are going to be fine, now you see clearly what you never saw before because of your former mad pace. Now all you need do is rely on the Great Cardiologist who, in His perfect love and wisdom, conferred on you the signal boon of a coronary occlusion to bring you to your senses.

Well, it will not be fine if you think that way, if you see even those truly valuable aspects of a heart attack—the enforced stock-taking and values-assessing—as anything other than the first tentative steps in the right direction.

Elmer Davis, probably the most scholarly and respected news commentator of his day, once responded to an article published in *Harper's* magazine that had been written as a prose version of Robert Browning's famous poem that begins "Grow old along with me/The best is yet to be." Davis wrote:

> . . . I am not persuaded that the best is yet to be, even by Catherine Drinker Bowen's eloquent disquisition in *Harper's* on the magnificence of age. . . . I cannot feel that the general public can draw much encouragement from the truly magnificent old age of the various worthies she mentions, notably Mr. Justice Oliver Wendell Holmes.
>
> It is no doubt true, as she says, that "luck being equal, whether a man at eighty finds himself reaping the harvest or the whirl-wind depends on how he has spent his forties and thirties and twenties." But luck is not equal; and it may be that to be an Oliver Wendell Holmes or a John Dewey at ninety you had to be a Holmes or a Dewey from the start, both in physical con-stitution and in potential mental capacity. . . . I have a friend aged eighty-four who is better than I am; but to judge from the record, she always was, at any age.

It is just the same with your husband's heart attack. Like growing old, it does nothing, by itself, for either of you. At least nothing that is particularly good, by itself. One Heart Wife told us that she had said to her husband, "I think you've been given a marvelous second chance. . . ." And so he had. And so had she. And so have you and your husband. But it is a second chance, an opportunity; it is not a sure thing, an automatic solution to your problems. A Holmes or a Dewey did not become great because he got old; indeed, he did not just "become" great at any age. He made himself great. You will not lead a better, saner, healthier life because your husband had a heart attack; but you can live a better, saner, healthier life—if you make it happen.

As we write this, the distinction seems so clear! How in the world could anyone think that the heart attack could be anything other than an opportunity that must be seized and exploited for everything it is worth, a suddenly ripe situation that must be squeezed of every drop that is in it if it is to be of the slightest benefit? Yet, having lived it, we know that the situation, living it day-by-day, is a good deal less clear.

A heart attack is so frightening and such a horrid experience and so everlastingly dreadful that once we can perceive the tiniest glimmer of good to come of it, we so easily shout hosannah and run toward the frail little suspicion of light as though it were the most glorious sunburst. It looks so bright—because it shines alone amid such gloom. And so it becomes such an easy matter to tell ourselves that, yes, it was for the best—because now look! how bright the future!

How bright indeed! That is the danger. It is not a false light we see when we contemplate the change in our husbands and ourselves. That shining hope for something better is real enough. But it is not enough. Because there is nothing of substance in the heart attack that automatically compels the right conclusion, let alone the right actions, from even the most searching reexamination of your goals, your values, or your lives. And without the fulfillment of possible benefits to the spirit of your marriage, the heart attack will leave the body of your marriage, like the body of your husband, distinctly weaker and less tenable.

In fact, that is an almost perfect analogy. Typically, a recovered heart patient is in dramatically better physical shape a year after the heart attack than he was a year before. His weight is down and so is his serum cholesterol; his muscle tone is better; his wind and stamina are much improved; he does not smoke, drink to excess, or get overtired (if he did any of those things before). Actually, his heart itself is stronger. But all that is because of what he did after the heart attack. The heart attack itself did nothing but give him a reason to live in a healthier manner.

Which brings you to the other fallacy, the "Worm in the Bud."

You must see the *non*-inevitability of improvement in order to be willing to bother working for improvement. So it is important to not look at a heart attack as some sort of automatic blessing. But it is equally important to not overcorrect on the other side. And that temptation is enormous, because it is so natural. The heart attack *is* terrible. It *is* scary. It *is* dangerous. And, yes, it *can* turn out horribly. As we said at the very beginning of the book, the most horrible and paralyzing aspect of a heart attack is the fact that if it happened before, it can happen again. No matter how careful your husband is, no matter how hard both of you try. The only answer to "Why me?" is . . . "Why not?" Again and again.

So what's the use?

Thinking that, you can easily take a "Worm in the Bud" attitude toward your life as a Heart Wife and as a cardiac couple. From the dangerous thought that, aha! a heart attack is automatically all for the best, you plunge into the equally damaging thought that it is inevitably all for the worst. You deny the possibility that anything about the life you see stretching bleakly before you can possibly be good or satisfying. How can anything be good when it derives from such an unrelieved horror as a heart attack! There will always be that worm, eating away at anything that looks like a flower in your life. Automatically So you refuse to take the slightest measure of comfort or joy from any potentially positive alternatives to a life of wretched despair. What's the use?

Both attitudes—mindless optimism or unthinking gloom—choke action with equal effectiveness.

The fact is, the heart attack is nothing. What you do about it is everything.

There is no area in the conduct of one's life where more depends directly on a person's own actions and attitude. Understand, we are not talking about the quality of your life in general; that still depends on all the factors that were operative before the heart attack, and will continue to be. But the difference in your husband's life, in your family's life, and in your life as a direct result of the heart attack, that difference depends almost exclusively on what you, your husband, and your family make of it.

We need not belabor the ways in which it can be bad—except to point out, again, that one of the quickest ways to assure a bad final result is to do nothing, to not take positive steps, rethinking your life and how it may have contributed to the attack.

But let's look at the good effects that flow from the conditions surrounding a patient's recovery from a heart attack, either absolutely, probably, or at least possibly.

— *Calm.* It is enforced at first and suggested forever. It may be a quite literal calm of resting and having time to think things over, or the more profound calm that can come to one's life as a result of such inward looking.

— *Reevaluation of goals.* Some reevaluation may be depressing, at least at first. If some of your goals as a person and as a couple now seem unlikely, impossible, or unwise, it may be hard to give them up. But in your reevaluation you are more likely to come to the same realization that so many Heart Wives have told us they and their husbands came to about "what is important and what is not."

— *Closeness.* There will be a new closeness between you and your husband because of the heart attack. There is the actual physical closeness, of course, of how many more hours you spend with him during early recovery. But, more important, there is the mental and spiritual closeness that comes of "peril shared." You are in this together from the first. And it does bring you closer together, as a team, than ever before.

— *Better understanding.* The need that you and your husband have to be concerned for each other with a rare selflessness will inevitably lead to a better understanding of each other's attitudes, wants, and needs.

And the greatest of these? Calm. It is the essential ingredient in all the other mixtures of the good life that can be the aftermath of the heart attack. Heart Wives have marveled over and over at how a sense of calm reflection bathes their lives with a warm, new appreciation for what there is to be derived from lives lived apart from a hectic worry about everything. The doctor discourages agonized turmoil over trifles as firmly as he discourages cholesterol. And calm is the saving grace of a heart attack; even if no other aspect of your husband's life improves, it will be of great benefit that, for a spell, he has had to be calm. With luck, it will become a permanent outlook for you both.

It is not at all too much to call it a blessing. Certainly it is the object of regular, formal prayer—perhaps best stated in a poem by John Greenleaf Whittier that, set to music, became a hymn:

> Dear Lord and Father of mankind,
> Forgive our foolish ways;
> Reclothe us in our rightful minds . . .
>
> Drop Thy still dews of quietness,
> Til' all our strivings cease;
> Take from our souls the strain and stress,
> And let our ordered lives confess,
> The beauty of Thy peace.
>
> Breathe through the heat of our desires
> Thy coolness and Thy balm;
> Let earth be still, let flesh retire;
> Speak through the earthquake, wind and fire,
> Thou still, small Voice of calm.

Perhaps the best way to illustrate that sense of calm, the realignment on your perspective of what is and is not important, is with a trivial example. It comes from a woman who is not a Heart Wife at all, but someone who herself had serious open-heart surgery. Talking with Mrs. D and her husband (who, we suppose, qualifies as a Heart Husband) gave us a fresh slant on the problems of a Heart Wife, since we could see the patient's attitude more clearly from the perspective of a woman. Mrs. D told us:

I used to be a compulsive cleaner, very uptight that there shouldn't be even a speck of dust anywhere around the house. Well, now I know that the cleaning isn't bad—but the being so uptight about it is what's bad. For me, and for my husband, too.

Now I'm too glad about being alive and enjoying it to worry about a little dust. And certainly not to get my husband all upset about it.

She said those words at a post-hospital meeting of cardiac couples. Others at the meeting were also speaking about the calm that had entered their lives:

MR. S: I'm really very, very content. I'm just happy. You can ask my wife; sometimes it gets her mad how happy I seem all the time, no matter what.

I get up in the morning happy; I go to bed at night happy. She tells me it's time to go to sleep, I go to sleep. I'm content to do whatever I'm doing!

MRS. D: I wonder if it isn't just being more conscious of it, being content.

You know, sometimes I wake up in the morning and the first thought that pops into my mind is, "I woke up this morning!"

I wake up very happy and very glad to be alive!

It's a very conscious thing with me, and I wonder how much of it is in you all the time—but you weren't really conscious of it before?

MRS. H: But my husband was always happy like that, even before.

MRS. D: Oh, then he won't change. He'll still be happy. He'll just know why—it's such a real joy to wake up in the morning. It's a beautiful thing—and it's *got* to be because of the heart attack!

You don't feel you have to push yourself anymore. You want to live and you're glad to be alive. You're feeling great, and you'll do what you're told by whoever

tells you if you think it's good for you, because it means
you're going to continue living longer.

The key is to concentrate on living. We asked another Heart
Wife whether the ever-present realization that her husband
might have another heart attack at any time, indeed might die at
any time—whether that did not constitute the Worm in the
Bud, the thought that turned all joy to ashes. She shook her head,
"No," and said:

MRS. P: I felt it was important for him to do what was important
    to him—even if I didn't approve or it worried me.
H.W.C.: Did you let it go at that?
MRS. P: Oh, no! You feel you want to help the man reevaluate.
    But this just doesn't happen overnight.

    I became philosophical. You have to! You can't live in
    a state of fear all the time. And it has to be a ...
    constructive fear or it's of no value. I had to do the things
    that would sustain him and try to make whatever time
    we had—a day or fifty years—as enjoyable as possible.
    To make our lives as interesting as possible and as
    worthwhile as I could.

    You have to do that while he's in the process of
    reevaluating things. Not dwelling on death as a pos-
    sibility, but on living. *Really* living. And that helps him
    make his own adjustments.

Some years ago the victim of a massive coronary thrombosis
wrote a book entitled *Thank God for My Heart Attack* (Holt,
Rinehart & Winston, 1949). In it, Charles Yale Harrison traced
exactly the mental progression that we are talking about.

But while we don't agree that there is reason to be "thankful"
for a heart attack, you certainly should give truly heartfelt
thanks if you can achieve as a result of your own attitude and
action, spurred by the heart attack, a new awareness, a new
sense of the worth of living. It is up to you.

You could not stop the heart attack from happening. You can do nothing to erase the scars on your husband's heart or expunge the physical damage of the heart attack. You can do nothing about the condition of the arteries that caused the heart attack in the first place, and might cause another some day. But you can do everything about the meaning of your husband's heart attack. You can control and shape that meaning. You can help decide if the meaning is to be one of good or evil for your life, your husband's life, and for your lives together.

Indeed, you can make a heart attack give a new meaning to both your lives for all the good years to come.

Index

Masculine self-image, in sexual activity, 243–44
Masculinity:
  assertion of, 102
  crisis, 201
  infringement on, 200
  and sexual needs, 230
McCuiston, Fred, xi, 25, 146
Meals, in bed, 216
Meal contents, 254
Meats, fat content, 267–68
Medical facts, 116–19
Medical judgment, wife's role in, 285
Medical treatment, resistance to, 100, 222
Medication:
  information about, 38
  neglect of, 200–1
  written record of, 147–48
Misbehavior, children's, 178–79
Monitor (*See* Cardiac monitor screen)
Mother, children's need for, 171
Mourning Becomes Electra (O'Neill), 245
Mouth-to-mouth resuscitation, 146
Myocardia infarct (*See* infarction)

N

Nagging, case history of, 224–25
Neglect, children's sense of, 174
Neutral Spirit, The (Roueché), 148
New England Journal of Medicine, 91
Noise, and children, 176–77
  at home, 143, 167
Notes, comparing between wives, 108–9
Nurses:
  behavior of, 129
  treatment of, 129–30
Nursing, at home, 143, 219–20

O

Observation Unit, Coronary Care Unit, 54–55
Oils, cooking, 264
Omega, xi
Oscilloscope screen, 54
Oxygen, need for, 11
Oxygen mask, 51
  positive breathing apparatus, 57
  supply of oxygen, Coronary Care Unit, 57

P

Patience, need for, 164
Personality change, 6–7, 95, 212
  during home recovery, 159–60
  in hospital, 101–3
  in hospital, example, 104–5
Pets, care of, 83, 181
Physical appearance, wife's, 77–78
Physiological changes, in hospital, 150–51
Pills, carrying of, 201
Pill box, use of, 148
Plaques, coronary, 12, 16
Polaroid camera, use of, 124
Polyunsaturated fats, defined, 262
Positive breathing apparatus, 57
Pregnancy, after husband's heart attack, 207–8
  case history, 210–11
Prinzmetal, Dr. Myron, 117
Problem-sharing, with children, 207
Progress reports, trading of, 109, 184–85
Psychological needs, in coronary recovery, 110–11

Q

Quarreling, cause of heart attack, 44–45

R

Rales, defined, 118
"Recipes for Fat-controlled, Low-cholesterol Meals," 120, 259
Recovery:
  children's role in, 166–67
  conditions for, 293–94
  at home, 151, 219–20
  hope for, 216
  period, length of, 33–34
Regime, recovery:
  atmosphere of, 191
  over-reaction to, 194
  wife's attitude toward, 191–92
Rehabilitation programs, state and county, 122
Relatives:
  children, care of, 79–80
  informing of attack, 62–64
    example, 63–65